ALSO BY EILEEN BEHAN, R.D.

MICROWAVE COOKING FOR YOUR
BABY AND CHILD

EAT WELL, LOSE WEIGHT WHILE BREASTFEEDING

EAT WELL, LOSE WEIGHT WHILE BREASTFEEDING

THE COMPLETE NUTRITION BOOK FOR NURSING MOTHERS, INCLUDING A HEALTHY GUIDE TO THE WEIGHT LOSS YOUR DOCTOR PROMISED

EILEEN BEHAN, R.D.

VILLARD BOOKS • NEW YORK

Library of Congress Cataloging-in-Publication Data

Behan, Eileen.
    Eat well, lose weight while breastfeeding : the complete nutrition book for nursing mothers, including a healthy guide to the weight loss your doctor promised / Eileen Behan.
        p.   cm.
    Includes bibliographical references and index.
    ISBN: 0-679-73355-8
    1. Breast feeding.   2. Mothers—Nutrition.   3. Lactation—Nutritional aspects.   4. Reducing diets.   I. Title.
RJ216.B34   1992
613.2′6—dc20   92-6324

Manufactured in the United States of America

B 9 8

In memory of my father, John Behan

To David, Sarah, and Emily.
We did it again. Thank you.

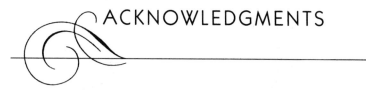

ACKNOWLEDGMENTS

To my mother, Sharon, Sheila, and Kevin, thanks for your continuous encouragement. Trish Cronan and Brad Lavigne, as always, you are a steadfast source of support. Judy Paige, Marilyn DeSimone, Madeleine Walsh, as friends and competent nutritionists, you continue to help me refine my ideas. I'd like to thank Ms. Ana Ortiz for efficient and accurate nutritional analysis of menus, and Susan Yorstin, thanks again for proofreading. Ms. Susan Cotter and Jennifer Quirk, thank you for your comments and development of the exercise program.

I would like to thank the following nutrition and lactation experts who generously gave their time to read all or part of this book before it went into print: Nancy F. Butte, Ph.D., Children's Nutrition Research Center, Houston, Texas; Bette Crase of the Center for Breastfeeding Information at La Leche League International; Kathryn Dewey, Ph.D., professor, Department of Nutrition, University of California, Davis, California; Lois Jovanovic-Peterson, M.D., senior scientist, Sansum Medical Research Foundation, Santa Barbara, California; Ruth A. Lawrence, M.D., professor of pediatrics, obstetrics, and gynecology, University of Rochester Medical Center, Rochester, New York; Susan Luke, M.S., R.D., nutritionist—sports medicine, Boston, Massachusetts; Arnold Schecter, M.D., professor of preventive medicine, State University of New York, Binghamton, New York.

At Villard Books I would like to thank Emily Bestler and her assistant, Tom Fiffer, for working patiently with me. I am also thankful to the others at Villard who contributed significantly to this book: Richard Aquan, Nancy Inglis, and Amy Ryan.

To Allison Acker and Carol Mann, once again you both saw the possibilities in my idea.

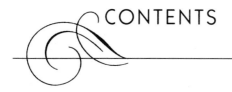

CONTENTS

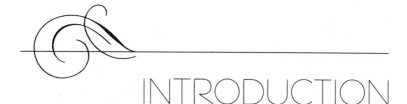

INTRODUCTION

"YOU SHOULD KNOW BETTER!" THOSE WERE MY DOCTOR'S WORDS as I sat in her office, nine months pregnant and weighing 187 pounds. She hadn't expected me to gain 52 pounds during my pregnancy. You see, I'm a registered dietitian, and food, nutrition, and diets are my business. But like many first-time moms I regarded pregnancy as a time to relax my eating standards. Almost every night I ate a bowl of delicious rich ice cream. I also snacked much more and found that if I didn't eat often I didn't have quite enough energy. In the beginning, food also helped fight nausea.

I really wasn't worried about my weight. I had always been able to maintain my weight between 130 and 135 pounds, which is fine for my 5'8" frame. I figured that after the baby was born, I would just get back to exercising and eating right and those excess pounds would melt away.

Three hours after my daughter Sarah was delivered by cesarean section, a food tray was brought to me. It carried coffee, red Jell-O, and chicken broth. These bland foods were supposed to restore my energy without taxing my digestive tract.

I hadn't eaten for more than eleven hours and I was hungry, but concerned. I contemplated the caffeine-, sodium-, and sugar-laden concoctions before me. Sure, they were safe for me, but what about when I breastfed Sarah? I realized that the foods I ate might pass into my breast milk and could upset or even harm her.

Because I would be nursing my daughter, my eating habits and occasional dietary indiscretions took on new significance. Should I drink coffee? Was the champagne that my husband and I planned to celebrate with safe? Were the pink-foil-wrapped chocolate cigars to be avoided? Could pesticides travel from the foods I ate into my breastmilk? How would fatty or cholesterol-rich foods affect Sarah? And what about my plans to lose weight? Could I breastfeed and lose weight too?

The hospital staff who were so competent at answering my husband's and my questions about breastfeeding techniques, baby baths, and diapering weren't well informed about diet. They told me, "Eat what you like; if it bothers the baby, then just avoid that food." But general recommendations weren't enough for the nutritionist in me. I wanted scientific studies to back up any eating decisions I made.

When I got home from the hospital, I looked through the breastfeeding and postpartum sections of my pregnancy books for answers to my nutrition questions. Unfortunately, their advice was just too vague: "Eat a balanced diet and avoid gassy food." There were no specific guidelines about how much coffee I could drink or information about the effects a glass of wine might have on the baby.

I was also advised not to worry about weight loss. Breastfeeding mothers are told they will automatically lose weight, even while eating the extra 500 calories a day recommended while nursing. In theory, these 500 calories, plus some taken from the mother's stored body fat, are used to make milk for the baby to thrive on. Well, I knew this wasn't entirely true. Studies have shown that breastfeeding mothers might not automatically lose weight if they follow this advice. Some mothers may require far fewer calories than the 2,700 per day recommended while nursing.

To answer my nutrition questions, I did my own research. I read all the respected lactation textbooks and talked to experts in the field. I developed a diet for myself that produced safe and gentle weight loss and kept my daughter Sarah happy, healthy, and in the ninetieth percentile for height and weight. When Sarah was nineteen months old, I was fortunate enough to have another happy, healthy little girl whom we named Emily. Once again I needed to lose weight, so I put my eating and nutrition plan into practice, and I was able to nurse my daughter, feel good, lose weight, and stay healthy and energetic.

This book is for all mothers who choose to breastfeed their children, but those of you concerned about the weight you gained during pregnancy will find it particularly helpful. Personally, I started to really worry about the way I looked and the rate at which I was losing weight about six weeks after Sarah was born. At that point, my daughter was thriving and I was confident about my ability to nurse, but I was still twenty-five pounds over my prepregnancy weight and had never been so tired in my life.

Not all of you will have reached the six-week postpartum stage. You brand-new moms shouldn't even begin to worry about losing weight until at least six weeks after delivery. You should just focus on taking care of yourself and your new baby. For those veteran moms ready to start losing weight, this book will give you the information you need to plan a sensible, gentle weight-loss program. Always keep in mind that your primary goal is to have a safe and satisfying nursing experience.

Some people say that new mothers shouldn't be forced to worry about losing weight because the challenges a new baby brings are all they should have to cope with. Being a sexy, skinny woman is an additional hassle they don't need. I absolutely agree. This book is not about trying to please someone else or about telling women they must look like the models in fashion magazines. A new mother is doing the most important job of her life. She should be proud of herself and not be apologetic about some excess bulge around her middle.

I've said it before and I'll keep saying it: While you are breast-feeding your primary job is to take care of yourself and your baby. It is not the time to be a supermom. Resist the pressure to jump right back into the rhythm of your previous life. You had a baby: whether it is your first or your fifth, take it easy on yourself.

But even if you decide that now is not the time to lose weight, it's still the perfect time to look critically at the food that passes over your family table. If your child hasn't started on food yet (and he shouldn't until he's four to six months old), he will eventually adopt the same eating patterns you have. If you eat lots of snacks or fried foods, then when your child is older and can make choices of his own, he'll eat the same way. So not only do you affect your own health by examining what you eat, you'll influence your child's health, too.

This book isn't just for mothers who want to lose weight; it's for any breastfeeding mom who wants to eat well. In chapter 1, you'll see why your decision to breastfeed is the right one. In chapters 2, 3, and 4, I'll explain how your body makes milk, how the food you eat affects your milk, and which nutrients are particularly important. In chapter 5, I'll discuss weight loss and how you can lose weight safely while breastfeeding.

In chapter 6, I'll show you a simple meal plan for weight loss that is safe for you and won't compromise your baby's health or your breastfeeding experience. In chapter 7, I'll talk about exercise—why it's important to set realistic goals for yourself and find a physical activity that you like. I'll also address the common reasons moms don't exercise and suggest ways for you to overcome those obstacles.

In chapter 8, I'll debunk some of those old wives' tales about foods like chocolate and cabbage upsetting the breastfeeding baby. I'll also discuss more serious concerns about pesticides, caffeine, nicotine, and alcohol passing into your breast milk and affecting your milk and your baby's health. Smart food choices can eliminate or minimize the risk these substances pose.

Mothers who have delivered by cesarean or who have health problems such as diabetes, anemia, or high blood pressure will have unique nutrition questions, which will be handled in chapter 9. In chapter 10, you'll find recipes to simplify your life. They are easy to prepare, made with familiar ingredients, and are nutritious, delicious, and freezable.

When I was a brand-new mom, I had tons of questions about nursing my baby. Sure, I knew about food, but nobody ever told me how to pick out a nursing bra that fit right or what to do if my breasts were engorged. In the final chapters, I've included a question-and-answer section as well as a list of excellent resources on breastfeeding and baby care.

I hope this book will give mothers enough information to make smart decisions about what to eat while they breastfeed, so they can feel good about themselves and their decision to nurse their babies. New mothers need to eat well so they'll have nutritious milk to feed their infants and the energy to care for them. My goal is to guide you to a healthy diet that will help you lose weight naturally and safely while you nourish a happy, healthy new child.

EAT WELL,
LOSE WEIGHT
WHILE
BREASTFEEDING

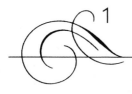 1

THE RIGHT
DECISION

THIS BOOK IS INTENDED TO HELP YOU EAT WELL, LOSE WEIGHT, and feel good about yourself, but that's not all it can do. I also want to support you in your decision to breastfeed your child so that you have a great nursing experience.

Breastfeeding is absolutely the best way to feed your baby, but American society is not always supportive of it. Before you begin reading about what to eat, I want you to appreciate that the feeding choice you made is a great one. I also want you to know that you aren't alone if you have some doubts about the choice you've made. Though breastfeeding is wonderful, it also has some drawbacks.

New mothers often doubt that they can breastfeed, even though it is the way nature meant for babies to be fed. Whatever you do, don't interpret these doubts to mean that you aren't capable of breastfeeding your baby. Even women who have had cesareans or twins or who have medical problems can nurse their children.

Take comfort in knowing that you are not the only mom who is fretful about her ability to breastfeed. Judy Jean Chapman, a nurse at Vanderbilt University, has studied what new mothers worry about. She found that when first starting to breastfeed, mothers worried most about having sore breasts, providing enough milk to feed their babies, and how frequently their babies nursed.

Of course the mothers also worried about the well-being of their babies. Fussiness, sleepiness, mixed-up days and nights, rashes, the rate of weight gain, and colds were the most frequently reported concerns. When the mothers were questioned about their own postpartum problems, fatigue topped the list. They also expressed concerns about their older children, returning to work or school, and the extra weight they still carried. I think anyone who has a frank discussion with a new nursing mom will hear some or all of these concerns. Of all the mothers I know, I can't think of one who approached breastfeeding with absolute confidence. Of course some women are more at ease right from the start, but for many mothers breastfeeding is a skill that must be learned and practiced before it becomes second nature.

If you're feeling overwhelmed by your worries, talk to a mother who has successfully breastfed her babies. If you don't have a friend you can speak to, call the experienced moms of the La Leche League. The national phone number is listed in the Resources section at the back of this book. You may also want to contact a lactation consultant, a woman who has special training in the subject of breastfeeding and who can assist you with almost any problem. See page 211 for information on how to locate a lactation consultant in your area.

IS BREAST REALLY BEST?

No matter how unsure you are about breastfeeding, you'll be happy to know that breastfeeding is the best way to nourish your baby. For your baby, it means getting the food that is perfectly designed to meet her nutrient needs. For you, it means losing weight and regaining your prepregnancy shape faster.

It is only in the twentieth century, with our sophisticated medical technology and research that we have to spend thousands, if not millions, of dollars on studies to prove what Mother Nature and you already know. Studies have shown that breastfeeding not only provides your baby with the ideal food, it also protects him against illness by passing some of your disease-fighting antibodies to him in your milk. Breastfed babies require fewer visits to the pediatrician than bottle-fed babies. This is true not only in third-world countries where disease is more prevalent, but in your household as well. A recent study on the protective effects of breastfeeding was conducted by Dr. Peter W. Howie and reported in the *British Medical Journal.* Dr. Howie studied more than six hundred Scottish mothers and their babies from birth to age two. He found that children who were nursed for at least thirteen weeks had significantly fewer reported incidences of vomiting and diarrhea than babies who were fed formula.

The protective effect of breastfeeding lasted even after breast milk stopped being a baby's main food. Babies who were nursed less than thirteen weeks seemed to have the same rate of vomiting and diarrhea as the formula-fed babies (while only vomiting and diarrhea were evaluated in this study, other reports show that breastfeeding protects against bronchitis, food poisoning, even influenza). The evidence from Dr. Howie's study points out that mothers should be actively encouraged by their doctors to breastfeed and to continue nursing for at least three months to get the maximum protection against disease for their babies.

Women who must return to work soon after delivery are also encouraged to breastfeed for at least the first three months. If a bottle of formula must be introduced, these mothers should try to use the bottle as a supplement and to keep breast milk as the primary food. Better yet, use expressed breast milk to fill that bottle.

Breastfed babies are not only healthier—they also have better teeth. According to Dr. Miriam H. Labbok of the Johns Hopkins School of Hygiene and Public Health, a breastfed baby will use her tongue to suck in a way that protects against misaligned teeth. Babies also use more muscles in their mouths when sucking from the breast, and this too protects against crooked teeth. This beneficial effect was found in children who were nursed for at least four months.

Breastfed babies are also less likely to get "nursing bottle syndrome." This happens when a child is left with a bottle in his mouth (usually while sleeping) and the liquid—be it milk, formula, or juice—pools around his tiny developing teeth, creating an ideal environment for cavities to form. A breastfed baby can't have a bottle propped up in his mouth while he falls asleep—he must be held while being fed. In addition, breastfed babies are less likely to suck their thumbs because breastfeeding allows them to satisfy their need to suck.

Another big plus is that you can't tamper with breast milk. Formula must be mixed or at the very least poured into bottles and consumed right away or stored and used within twenty-four hours. At any of these preparation stages, it is possible to contaminate the formula. Breast milk comes out of the breast safe and ready to serve. Some formulas that require the addition of water can be over- or underdiluted, while breast milk is created in the perfect concentration.

Breast milk is even tailored to the baby's age and nutritional needs. Breast milk is rich in protein at the beginning of a feeding, while the end of the feeding contains more fat, the nutrient that provides lots of good calories and assuages hunger pangs. Mothers of premature babies produce milk that is richer in protein than the milk of mothers of full-term babies. As the premature baby grows, the composition of the mother's milk changes automatically to meet the baby's needs. Within one month, it becomes the same as full-term milk.

Another fact to keep in mind is that the breastfeeding mom can't regulate how much her baby eats. A breastfeeding baby drinks exactly as much or as little milk as she wants, and this is good thing, because only the baby really knows how much she needs. Mothers and baby-sitters who see that the baby has drunk only half a bottle may feel compelled to make the baby finish that bottle, even though she doesn't really want it or need it, setting the stage for potential eating or weight problems down the road.

Is Your Baby Getting Enough to Eat?

Some breastfeeding moms worry that since they can't see how much their babies drink, they might not be drinking enough. A newborn baby who wets six or more diapers every day, has two to five bowel movements, has six to ten feedings, looks and acts healthy, and is gaining weight is sure to be getting enough breast milk.

Once you and your baby become a "nursing couple," you'll quickly discover some of the secondary benefits of breastfeeding. A baby cradled in his mother's arms and nursing at her breast must be the most secure being on earth. He's comforted by the warm skin-to-skin contact. If he glances upward, his twelve- to fifteen-inch visual range clearly captures his mom's smile and loving eyes. This experience goes a long way toward providing your child with a sound emotional foundation for life.

Your decision to breastfeed has some purely selfish benefits too. Because you're breastfeeding, you'll have to sit down and put your feet up throughout the day as you nurse your baby. Very small infants may need to nurse every one to two hours, and a ten-month-old may nurse three to five times a day. While the baby eats you really can't do much else, which means that you get a little rest, too.

Breastfeeding can also help the family budget, since you won't have to buy expensive cans of formula. You can save an average of $100 a month, which adds up to $1,200 in a year.

If you had iron-deficiency anemia while pregnant, breastfeeding may help you conserve iron. Breastfeeding often stops menstruation for six to twelve months after you give birth, which means you won't be losing the iron normally lost with menstrual bleeding. This temporary cessation of menstruation also reduces your chance of getting pregnant, but please don't count on breastfeeding as a means of birth control—it isn't reliable.

Breastfeeding also helps your body get back in shape. Because your body is making milk for your child, you'll need extra calories, some of which will come from the fat you stored during pregnancy. Breastfeeding also causes your uterus to contract, and this can help return your tummy to its prepregnancy shape sooner.

Besides the benefits to you and your baby, breastfeeding can help Mother Earth. You won't be using disposable bottles or bottle liners or plastic bottles or adding empty formula cans to overflowing landfills. This will have only a small impact on the environment, but it is another way you can protect your baby's future.

SOME CHALLENGES OF BREASTFEEDING

Breastfeeding is not without problems. As I mentioned earlier, you're likely to find it stressful at times. Since you are your child's sole source of food, you won't be able to leave her easily for any extended time. In emergencies, or if you plan ahead, you can express a supply of milk and keep it in the freezer until needed. But when your baby wakes up at 1:00 A.M., 3:00 A.M., and 5:00 A.M. it's you she wants. Sure, many dads help by getting up and bringing the baby to mom, but then they get to go back to sleep. You're on duty.

At social events it's often the mother who provides most of the care. In the beginning, when little babies cry unpredictably, the breast is one of the surefire ways to calm them down. If you aren't completely at ease with nursing in public, this will mean finding quiet, out-of-the-way places to nurse and missing out on some of the activities.

When my daughter Sarah was a newborn, my husband and I were taking a course in Boston. I could never breastfeed comfortably among strangers. I found myself spending most of my class time in a corner of the ladies' room that fortunately had a comfortable seat. And I remember taking Sarah on her first airplane ride when she was ten weeks old. The plane was packed with businessmen, there were no empty seats, and the aisle seat I had requested was taken. I had no elbow room to breastfeed, so I spent a good deal of the flight in the airplane's restroom nursing Sarah.

There is another side to breastfeeding that most of us veterans don't like to share with new moms because it may be discouraging. Breastfed babies don't sleep the way bottle-fed babies do. In fact, they usually sleep less and wake more often.

The "normal" (if there really is such a thing) nighttime sleep cycle for newborns is about four to five hours long, which stretches to eight to ten hours by the third or fourth month. In all, the "normal" infant sleeps thirteen to fifteen hours out of every twenty-four; this decreases only slightly by the second birthday.

If you can get your child to sleep those eight to ten hours at night and all at once, then the two of you can get some much-needed rest. Unfortunately, breastfed babies don't often sleep for such long stretches. When Dr. Marjorie F. Elias of Harvard University decided to study the sleep patterns of breastfed babies, she found that breastfed babies didn't consistently sleep for eight to ten unbroken hours until the second year, usually after they were weaned. Those infants who shared a bed with their mothers had even shorter stretches of sleep than babies in cribs.

I share this information with you to let you know that you aren't alone if you're worried about your child's sleep patterns. Lack of sleep is a big source of concern to mothers. If you're feeling tired and more worn out than ever, you have good reason. Don't be discouraged. Instead, set your priorities. Take care of yourself and your baby. If you can't keep up with the housework, don't be alarmed. Do what you can. You can always do the rest later. What you can't get back is this precious time with your child.

Well-meaning friends will give you all sorts of advice about getting your child to sleep. They'll tell you to introduce solid food early, let your child cry it out, or wean your child. Don't be pressured into doing anything that doesn't feel right to you. If you're really worried about your baby's behavior or health, talk to your doctor, other breastfeeding moms, the La Leche League, or a good lactation consultant.

Take comfort in knowing that it is normal for newborns to be wakeful, and normal for mothers to have a hard time adjusting to their babies' schedules. I wasn't able to count on either of my girls sleeping through the night until they were about fifteen months old. This might sound ghastly to you, but it wasn't bad. I really got used to it and came to enjoy our quiet time together. After their first birthdays they would usually wake up only once in the night, and I think that was more for reassurance than anything else. Today four-year-old Sarah and two-year-old Emily are champion sleepers. I have a secret theory that infants who wake frequently as babies and are comforted by their moms or dads grow up to be sound sleepers.

NEW MOTHERS NEED SUPPORT

Our culture isn't always supportive of mothering or of breastfeeding. Many women must return to full-time jobs while their babies are young, and they worry whether or not they'll be able to combine nursing and work. Or their families may not understand why a mother would choose to breastfeed when she can formula feed.

According to a report in the *Medical Tribune,* a national survey found that 70 percent of mothers having a baby today would want to breastfeed and that 80 percent of the men asked would support their mates' decision to breastfeed. But despite the desire to nurse, the rate of breastfeeding in the United States is declining for all ages and socioeconomic groups.

In the 1930s, about 70 percent of babies were breastfed; by 1960, that number plunged to 30 percent. The decline in the 1960s was probably the result of the introduction and mass marketing of baby formula. In the 1970s, there was a strong countertrend, and more mothers returned to nursing. But the late 1980s saw a gradual decline in breastfeeding. A 1990 study conducted by Ross Laboratories found that 51.4 percent of all babies were breastfed while in the hospital. That's down from 58 percent in 1985.

Statistics from the U.S. Bureau of the Census indicate that in 1988 (the most recent year for which data are available) 52 percent of married women with children less than one year of age were working outside the home. Returning to work is often used as a reason for stopping breastfeeding and in some cases not even starting it. The statistics point out that we need to be more supportive of mothers and children in this country. Mothers need longer maternity leave, adequate facilities for feeding their children at work, and on-site, affordable childcare if we are to reverse the disturbing trend away from breastfeeding.

Your breastfed child is very lucky. In the long run you won't regret any inconvenience, and your child will be happier and healthier because of it. Breastfeeding is likely to be the first important decision you make about your baby's health and upbringing. It's one of the few parenting decisions that is unanimously recognized as being the right one. Breast truly is best.

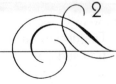

THEY ARE
WHAT YOU EAT

LACTATION IS THE NATURAL CONTINUATION OF YOUR PREG-nancy. Look upon pregnancy as an eighteen-month experience. The first nine months are for building the baby, the next nine for breastfeeding her. Of course, many mothers breastfeed for much longer than nine months. However long you choose to nurse, it's important that you remember to take just as good care of yourself after you have the baby as you did while you were pregnant. Good care includes good eating.

Diet plays as big a role in lactation as it does in pregnancy. The nutrients you stored and those you eat every day will be what nourishes your baby. At no other time in your life will there be such a demand on your physical resources. If this sounds intimidating, don't fret. Your only job is to provide your body with nutritious food. It will then efficiently and elegantly trans-form that food into a perfectly balanced blend of nutrients for your baby.

HOW THE BREAST MAKES MILK

During your pregnancy, you no doubt noticed changes in your breasts; they got larger, became tender, and the nipples and areolae (the area around the nipples) darkened. These temporary changes occur in preparation for breastfeeding.

The milk sacs, or alveoli, in your breasts are stimulated by the hormones your body creates during pregnancy; by the second trimester these alveoli can produce early milk, which could help feed a baby born prematurely. Within twenty-four hours of birth, the hormones in your body change again, this time signaling full-scale milk production to begin. These physical and hormonal changes, combined with the stimulation provided by the baby's sucking at the breast, will allow for steady and regular milk production.

The yellow colostrum is the first milk your breasts make. It is extremely rich in protein and carries important disease-fighting antibodies essential to a newborn's health. Colostrum is replaced by true milk a couple of days after delivery. As long as the baby is allowed to feed regularly at the breast, your body will automatically produce an adequate supply of milk, even if you are nursing twins or triplets.

Your breasts increase in size during the time you breastfeed because of the extra blood flowing through them. The blood carries nutrients from your digestive tract to the breast and eventually to your baby. Prepregnancy breast size has nothing to do with a woman's ability to nurse successfully. All women have the same milk-producing equipment. Women with large breasts simply have more fat tissue surrounding the milk-making apparatus.

WHO WILL SUFFER IF MOM'S DIET ISN'T NUTRITIOUS?

The good news is that even if your diet is less than ideal, your body is still able to manufacture nourishing breast milk. This is

Mother Nature's way of insuring that your baby is well fed. In most cases a mother would have to eat an extremely restricted diet for a long time to create a nutritional deficiency in her breast milk. This can happen, but fortunately it's rare.

However, a diet inadequate in calories and nutrients will have some negative effects. Mothers who can't or won't eat enough good, healthy food are more likely to feel tired and irritable. When combined with the fatigue from caring for a new baby, this adds up to a less than ideal nursing situation. Since fatigue is one of the main reasons women stop nursing, it's vital to eat well to keep your stamina up.

A diet inadequate in calories can decrease breast-milk production. One skipped meal won't matter, but mothers who never quite get enough to eat because they are dieting, have self-imposed food restrictions, or just can't afford enough food can produce smaller quantities of milk. You can just guess what happens when milk production drops: babies become hungry and very cranky.

Calories are one factor in your diet, nutrients are another. If a mother's diet lacks a nutrient, then that nutrient will be pulled from the supply stored in her body. In this way, breast milk contains a constant supply of nutrients despite day-to-day fluctuations in what the mother eats. This drain on a mom's reserves isn't harmful as long as she keeps those supplies replenished by eating a variety of nutritious foods. If these reserves aren't replaced, then the mother could suffer long-term negative health consequences.

HOW DO YOU KNOW IF YOUR BABY IS EATING ENOUGH?

A newborn baby who feeds about ten times a day at the breast and wets six or more diapers every day is probably getting plenty to eat. Weight checks conducted by your doctor will also be a good guide. Your child will be weighed and measured at the two-week, two-month, and four-month doctor's visit. Checking weight at home is not recommended because it puts too much emphasis on the scale, and home scales are often inaccurate. Instead, pay attention to your baby's moods. If he appears bright, alert, and happy most of the time, then chances are very good that he is healthy and eating enough.

If you're worried about how often your baby nurses, you aren't alone. Listen to a group of new mothers and you are sure to hear them talk about their feeding worries, such as how often baby feeds, falls asleep at the breast, fusses, or even refuses to eat. Do these concerns sound familiar? Don't suffer silently. Talk to your pediatrician or her staff, talk to another mother who is breast-feeding, or call the La Leche League. Support during the first few weeks is very important to new moms, so seek it out. When Sarah was six weeks old we joined a mothers' group of five mothers. A mothers' group is one of the few places you can talk about babies, babies, babies and not bore everyone to death. Hearing about their problems can help reassure you that you're not alone.

Many mothers comment that their breast milk looks too thin and watery; they worry that it isn't rich enough to nourish their babies. This isn't true. Breast milk is the ideal food for newborns. It may appear thin when compared to cow's milk, but it is loaded with the nutrients your baby needs.

It's very hard for new mothers to breastfeed when other family members aren't supportive. Older family members may make comments like "You're starving that baby by giving him just breast milk—give him formula or cereal too." If this happens to you, look for outside support. Try to find another experienced mom who can give you advice and comfort, or contact the La Leche League.

Try not to worry about starting solid foods for the first few months. Most doctors currently recommend that mothers not introduce solid foods to their babies for at least four months. What most of us forget is that breast milk is food—it's just in liquid form. It's perfectly balanced in protein and all the other nutrients that your baby needs.

SHOULD I TAKE A MULTIVITAMIN?

Breastfeeding moms are encouraged to get their nutrition from food, not supplements. Food is simply the most reliable and direct way to get the nutrients you need. A proper diet makes supplements redundant. An orange doesn't contain just vitamin C. It has health-promoting fiber and is a delicious form of energy-providing carbohydrate. A vitamin C tablet contains only vitamin C, with some sort of filler and no energy or fiber. It's not uncommon for mothers to continue prenatal vitamins while they nurse. This is fine, but don't expect a vitamin tablet to replace good healthy food.

However, some breastfeeding mothers really do need to take supplements. A breastfeeding mother who is getting 1,800 calories a day or less will need a balanced multivitamin-mineral supplement because the volume of food she is eating is just too low to meet her nutritional needs. Mothers who are vegetarians and avoid all the animal foods that carry vitamin B_{12} will need to take a B_{12} supplement (2.6 micrograms per day). If a mother isn't eating milk, cheese, or other calcium-rich dairy products, she'll need a calcium supplement. Mothers who avoid vitamin D–fortified food such as milk or cereal and have little exposure to sunlight may be in need of a vitamin D supplement. All these mothers should seek out advice from a physician or nutrition counselor.

HOW DO I CHOOSE A SUPPLEMENT?

Supplements available by prescription and designed for new mothers are good and reliable but often more expensive than an equally good over-the-counter multivitamin. When selecting a supplement to "round out" your menu, look for one that contains both vitamins and minerals. Read the label. It will contain a list of the nutrients included and the percentage of the recommended dietary allowances (RDAs) that they provide. A good supplement to choose while breastfeeding is one that contains all or most of the nutrients listed on page 21. Calcium, zinc, magnesium, vitamin B_6, and folic acid (folate) should be included, because some mothers don't get enough of these nutrients. Supplements should not exceed the recommended levels based on the RDAs; when taken in excessive amounts, some nutrients can interfere with the absorption of others.

ARE THERE ANY NUTRIENTS I SHOULD BE CAREFUL ABOUT WHILE NURSING?

There are a few nutrients that if taken in doses that greatly exceed the RDA could increase the content of this nutrient in your breast milk to an undesirable level. These include vitamin B_6, vitamin D, iodine, and selenium. There are no studies to document whether these nutrients could become toxic to your baby, but who wants to take a chance? Be safe and don't take excessive amounts of any of these nutrients.

WILL A MULTIVITAMIN BOOST THE NUTRITIONAL CONTENT OF MY BREAST MILK?

The notion of increasing the nutrients in your milk by taking a multivitamin might have a certain appeal and might even sound logical. Unfortunately, it won't work.

Mothers who are already well nourished won't increase the nutritional quality of their milk by taking multivitamins. Dr. M. Rita Thomas, a researcher specializing in the nutrition needs of breastfeeding mothers, studied the effect supplements had on well-nourished women who had been nursing for six months. She specifically examined the quantities of vitamin C, vitamin B_6, vitamin B_{12}, folic acid, riboflavin, and thiamine found in their breast milk. She found that the vitamin supplements did not affect the nutrient concentration of the breast milk. Please notice that the women studied were already well nourished. Women who have diets that are only marginally adequate and are undernourished themselves *can* increase the nutritional quality of their breast milk by taking supplements.

What you eat while breastfeeding matters. The mother who takes time to eat well will be doing herself and her baby a favor. Don't rely on vitamin and mineral pills alone to provide you with nourishment. Eat health-promoting foods like fruits, vegetables, low-fat protein sources, whole grains, and dairy products and your body will be perfectly prepared to make the milk your child will thrive upon.

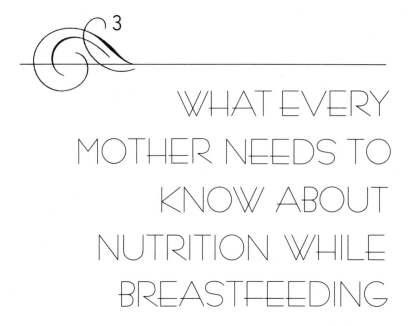

WHAT EVERY MOTHER NEEDS TO KNOW ABOUT NUTRITION WHILE BREASTFEEDING

THIS CHAPTER IS ABOUT HELPING MOTHERS MAKE SMART CHOICES. Gross nutritional deficiencies are unlikely for most nursing mothers in America, but subtle nutrient inadequacies may be a problem. I know from talking to many clients that not everyone is sitting down to three balanced meals a day. I also know that new mothers have a hard time trying to feed themselves and keep up with all their other commitments. The good news is that women who eat conventional diets that include a wide variety of foods are extremely unlikely to have serious nutrition problems. Most nutrients are not difficult to get if smart food choices are made. Even if a mother falls a bit short of meeting the recommended dietary allowances (RDAs), there is likely to be little impact on her breast milk.

For years the nutritional recommendations for nursing mothers have been quite general: "Eat a little more of all the food groups and you'll do fine." This is not bad advice; it's just not very specific. Some mothers need to learn more about nutrition and change their diets so that they get enough of the foods they really do need. For instance, the levels of selenium and iodine in your breast milk are dependent on how much of these nutrients you eat. If you take supplements, large doses of nutrients such as vitamin B_6, vitamin D, iodine, and selenium might increase the levels of these nutrients in your breast milk to a point that could be detrimental to your baby.

While you are nursing, your need for calcium, magnesium, zinc, folic acid, and vitamin B_6 goes up dramatically, and it's important to select foods rich in these nutrients. It is particularly vital for you to pay attention to the amount of calcium and folic acid you consume, since these nutrients will be kept constant in breast milk at your expense. It is not yet known for sure, but mothers who don't get enough calcium while nursing may be at greater risk for developing osteoporosis when they get older.

Recognizable deficiencies of thiamine, vitamin B_6, biotin, vitamin B_{12}, and vitamins D and K have been found in breastfeeding mothers who weren't eating enough of the foods they needed. These deficiencies have occurred in mothers in third-world countries where food was simply not available. When deficiencies in babies as well as mothers have occurred in the United States they have been the result of extremely rigid, restricted diets that mostly consisted of vegetables. Some of the more dramatic cases in this country have occurred with vitamin D and vitamin B_{12} deficiencies. This may sound alarming, but in truth a mother will not be able to create a nutritional deficiency in her baby unless her diet is extremely limited.

Nutritional requirements are different for women of childbearing age and for pregnant and lactating women (table 1). Some requirements for breastfeeding women, such as that for protein, can be easily met, while other requirements, such as those for zinc, iron, and calcium, are often inadequate in the diet of new mothers. Breastfeeding creates unique demands on your body, and a few nutrients are particularly critical while you're nursing (table 2). These nutrients are either hard to get, extremely important to mother or baby, or potentially harmful if taken in excessive amounts.

Table 1. Just What a Woman Needs

These recommendations assume a woman is in good health and moderately active. Adolescents may have greater nutritional needs, since they may still be growing during pregnancy and lactation.

Nutrient	Women 25–50	Pregnant	Lactating (0–6 months)	Lactating (6–12 months)
Protein	50 g	60 g	65 g	62 g
Vitamin A	800 mcg RE	800 mcg RE	1,300 mcg RE	1,200 mcg RE
Vitamin D	5 mcg	10 mcg	10 mcg	10 mcg
Vitamin E	8 mg	10 mg	12 mg	11 mg
Vitamin K	65 mcg	65 mcg	65 mcg	65 mcg
Vitamin C	60 mg	70 mg	95 mg	90 mg
Thiamine	1.1 mg	1.5 mg	1.6 mg	1.6 mg
Riboflavin	1.3 mg	1.6 mg	1.8 mg	1.7 mg
Niacin	15 mg	17 mg	20 mg	20 mg
Vitamin B_6	1.6 mg	2.2 mg	2.1 mg	2.1 mg
Folic Acid	180 mcg	400 mcg	280 mcg	260 mcg
Vitamin B_{12}	2.0 mcg	2.2 mcg	2.6 mcg	2.6 mcg
Calcium	800 mg	1,200 mg	1,200 mg	1,200 mg
Phosphorus	800 mg	1,200 mg	1,200 mg	1,200 mg
Magnesium	280 mg	320 mg	355 mg	340 mg
Iron	15 mg	30 mg	15 mg	15 mg
Zinc	12 mg	15 mg	19 mg	16 mg
Iodine	150 mcg	175 mcg	200 mcg	200 mcg
Selenium	55 mcg	65 mcg	75 mcg	75 mcg

Some of these numbers might vary from those you see on labels. Labels carry the U.S. RDA. These are numbers for healthy adult men and women. While breastfeeding, the RDA for all nutrients increases, hence the variation. Notice too that vitamin A and vitamin E are no longer measured in international units (IU). The new measurements, which are thought to be more accurate, are in mcg RE (Retinol equivalents) for vitamin A and mg for vitamin E.

Most of a woman's nutrient requirements increase steadily with the demands of pregnancy and early lactation. By the second six months of lactation, a baby is getting more of his nourishment from solid foods and less from breast milk, which decreases the nutrients needed by his mother.

Table 2. Critical Nutrients for Breastfeeding Women

Nutrients That Are Most Often Deficient

Calcium	Vitamin B_6
Zinc	Folic Acid
Magnesium	

Nutrients Difficult to Obtain on Low-Calorie or Restricted Diets

Calcium	Iron
Zinc	Vitamin E
Magnesium	Riboflavin
Vitamin B_6	Selenium (possibly)
Folic Acid	Niacin (possibly)
Thiamine	

Nutrients Easily Obtained from Conventional Diets

Protein	Vitamin A
Fat	Vitamin D
Sodium	Vitamin K
Potassium	Vitamin B_{12}
Copper	Biotin
Vitamin C	Iodine
Pantothenic Acid	Manganese
Fluoride	Chromium
Molybdenum	

Nutrients That Might Be Harmful if Overconsumed as Supplements

Vitamin B_6	Iodine
Vitamin D	Selenium

VITAL NUTRIENTS FOR THE BREASTFEEDING MOTHER

To help you evaluate your diet and plan healthy menus, I'll discuss every major nutrient on the following pages, explaining the role each plays in promoting good health. Keep in mind that nutrients have the same health-promoting effect for your baby as they do for you. The recommendations given here are based on the U.S. recommended dietary allowances established for breast-feeding mothers.

Protein

Protein is your body's basic building material. Muscles, organs, bones, cartilage, skin, antibodies, enzymes, and some hormones are all made from protein. You need it and so does your baby. Each day, a nursing mother secretes about 6 to 11 grams of protein in her breast milk to nourish her baby. A breastfeeding mother needs an extra 12 to 15 grams of protein each day to meet the protein needs of her and her baby. Two extra glasses of milk or two extra eggs at breakfast can meet this demand.

In most cases, getting adequate protein is not difficult, providing you eat foods like eggs, beef, chicken, and milk. In a study of middle-class American breastfeeding mothers, it was found that these women ate, on average, 94 grams of protein a day, significantly more than the recommended intake of 65 grams. Vegetarians need to pay more attention to their protein intake, but they can easily get enough of this nutrient by making intelligent food choices (read about the vegetarian diet in chapter 9). A glass of milk provides 8 grams of protein, one egg contains 7 grams, and a cup of cooked beans will provide a mother with 13 grams.

We can't store protein as we do some other nutrients, so we need a new supply every day. Protein deficiency is most likely to become a problem when budgets get tight. Protein-rich foods like beef, chicken, and fish are expensive. If a mother isn't able to eat the recommended amount of protein, the protein for her baby will be drawn from the mother's muscle tissue, sapping the mother's strength and even increasing her chances for illness.

Many of the protein-rich foods I've listed contain other vital nutrients, such as zinc and iron. Unfortunately, protein-rich animal foods also contain cholesterol and saturated fats. You can reduce the fat by trimming your meats and removing the skin from poultry before eating it and by choosing low-fat dairy products.

Some experts believe that eating too much protein interferes with the body's calcium balance, thus increasing our risk of osteoporosis as we get older. Excessive intake of protein may also be connected with kidney disease in old age, perhaps because the kidneys become overworked from trying to eliminate excessive by-products of protein digestion.

Protein is very important for nursing mothers, but don't overdo it. You can get too much of a good thing. A nursing mother needs at least 7 ounces of meat, fish, chicken, or protein alternative (dairy foods or properly combined portions of beans, nuts, and grains) each day. Unless a mother is extremely active, she probably won't ever need more than 8 or 9 ounces of these foods to meet the protein needs of her and her nursing baby.

Good sources of protein: chicken, beef, fish, turkey, cheese, eggs, milk, yogurt, grains (oatmeal, brown rice, pasta, whole-wheat bread), and legumes and nuts (peanuts, cashews, almonds, lentils, soybeans, kidney beans, tofu). Grains, legumes, and nuts all contain incomplete protein. That means they carry only some of the essential amino acids that your body needs to make its own protein. Incomplete protein foods must be combined with each other to make a complete protein. Meat, fish, poultry, and dairy products contain all the essential amino acids your body needs and are referred to as complete proteins.

Even if you don't eat much meat, a small amount of animal protein such as a few ounces of hamburger or ground turkey scrambled into a spaghetti sauce significantly boosts the protein value of a meal.

Vitamin A

Vitamin A does much more than promote good vision. It keeps skin healthy, helps make some essential hormones, assists the immune system, and even helps make red blood cells.

A healthy American mother passes about 400 to 670 micrograms of vitamin A each day to her baby through her breast milk. A nursing mom must consume an extra 400 to 500 micrograms of vitamin A each day, for a total of 1,300 micrograms daily. The mother's need for vitamin A drops a bit in the second six months of nursing to 1,200 micrograms, since the baby starts to get more nutrients from solid foods.

Women in wealthy industrialized nations like the United States are unlikely to be vitamin-A deficient or produce vitamin-A deficient milk. Mother Nature recognizes the importance of vitamin A and arms the female body with enough storage capacity to prevent deficiencies. Well-nourished mothers usually have about 200 milligrams of vitamin A stored in their bodies. A baby who breastfeeds exclusively for the first six months and then partially until the first birthday will consume about 192 milligrams of vitamin A. Even if a mother didn't eat any food containing vitamin A (which would be extremely difficult, if not impossible to do), her breastfeeding baby would still not entirely deplete his mother's stores of vitamin A.

Vitamin A is fat-soluble, which means the body stores any excess in fat tissue. Toxic reactions can occur if supplements are used at amounts that far exceed the RDA. These toxic reactions can include headache, vomiting, and liver damage. Mothers who take extremely large doses of vitamin A run the risk of increasing the vitamin A content of their breast milk to an unhealthy level.

Good sources of vitamin A: liver, eggs, milk, sweet potato, carrot, spinach, winter squash, greens, cantaloupe, mango, papaya, tomato, and apricot.

Deep orange, green, or red foods are usually very good sources of vitamin A, as are most fruits and vegetables. Studies have found that the vitamin A content of breast milk actually increases in spring and summer when we eat more vitamin A–rich produce.

Vitamin D

Vitamin D builds strong bones for both you and your baby by working with calcium and phosphorus to harden or mineralize bones. Vitamin D deficiency can cause rickets, a disorder in which bones don't form properly. In parts of the world where people don't or can't consume enough vitamin D, children develop rickety bowed legs when they start to walk. Their soft bones are so weak that they bow under the child's weight. Fortunately, rickets is quite rare in the United States.

We can get our vitamin D from food and supplements, or our bodies can manufacture it when we're exposed to sunlight. The RDA for vitamin D for a pregnant and nursing mother is 10 micrograms, double the amount required by a nonpregnant woman. A baby will consume only about 0.3 to 0.6 micrograms in a full day's supply of breast milk. That leaves a lot of vitamin D to meet the needs of the mother. Much of this extra vitamin D works with calcium to maintain the mother's good health. Vitamin D deficiences have only been found in breastfed babies born to mothers who ate diets completely lacking vitamin D and who also limited their babies' exposure to sunlight.

Sunlight converts vitamin D precursors in the body into the real thing. Your baby can get a week's supply of vitamin D by spending two hours outside without a hat or thirty minutes in the sun wearing just a diaper. Babies with dark skin may need slightly longer exposure. If you don't get out in the sun much, your pediatrician may recommend a vitamin D supplement for your baby. Because I lived in the Northeast, where winters sometimes seem to go on forever and days at the beach are really limited, my pediatrician prescribed a vitamin supplement with vitamin D. Moms living in southern California or sunny Florida shouldn't have to worry about such things.

Don't start self-prescribing large quantities of vitamin D for you or your baby. If you take too much of this vitamin, potentially toxic amounts can be secreted into your breast milk. Supplements that exceed the RDA levels are not advised. Talk to your pediatrician before giving your baby vitamin D supplements.

Good sources of vitamin D: vitamin D–fortified milk (one cup supplies about 25 percent of the vitamin D needed by adults), vitamin D–fortified margarine, eggs, liver, and fish. There are no reliable plant sources of this nutrient.

Vitamin E

Vitamin E helps protect the muscles, cardiovascular system, and nerve membranes from the damaging reactions that are a normal part of metabolism. It also helps the body use vitamin A. Vitamin E deficiency can show up as a certain type of anemia or as a degeneration and weakness of the muscles.

In the first six months of breastfeeding, a mother's need for vitamin E is thought to increase by at least 3 milligrams a day. The RDA for vitamin E is set higher than the amount you'll actually need because your body may not efficiently absorb this nutrient from food. Your baby will be taking in 1.4 to 2.3 milligrams of vitamin E in the breast milk he drinks every day. To meet your own needs for vitamin E and the needs of your nursing baby, the RDA is set at 12 milligrams. This drops to 11 milligrams in the second six months of breastfeeding, when the nutrient demands on your body lessen somewhat.

Colostrum, the first milk your baby drinks, is extremely rich in vitamin E. In the first days of life, your baby will more than triple his own blood levels of this nutrient. A 1977 study found that unless supplements were given to formula-fed babies, they had chronically low levels of vitamin E in the first six months of life.

Your own vitamin E intake may not meet the RDA unless you select food wisely and eat enough calories. It has been estimated that a mother eating only 1,800 calories may ingest only 9 of 11 to 12 milligrams of vitamin E needed each day.

One study reports that a mother consuming 27 milligrams per day of vitamin E increased the vitamin E concentration in her breast milk to 11 milligrams per liter (the usual concentration is 2.3 milligrams per liter). This increase is quite significant; since no one knows what effect this might have on a developing baby, the use of large doses of vitamin E while breastfeeding is not recommended.

Good sources of vitamin E: plant oils (corn oil, vegetable oil, margarine), salad dressing, wheat germ, butter, liver, egg yolk, nuts, seeds, and green leafy vegetables.

Vitamin K

Vitamin K is called the blood clotting nutrient in honor of its most important function. A woman's requirements for vitamin K are not thought to increase during pregnancy or lactation. Vitamin K is so abundant in food that adult women get much more than they actually need. The RDA is set at 65 micrograms daily; only 1.3 to 2.1 micrograms are secreted into breast milk. Even though a mother may eat adequate amounts of this nutrient, breast milk is naturally low in vitamin K. A liter of breast milk contains only 2 micrograms, while an equal amount of formula fortified with vitamin K contains over 20 micrograms.

All babies have to develop the ability to clot blood, which makes them immediately dependent on an external source of vitamin K. Even thriving newborns can develop a hemorrhaging syndrome caused by vitamin K deficiency. To prevent this potentially lethal condition, the American Academy of Pediatrics recommends that all newborns get a one-time injection of vitamin K, which is administered soon after birth and takes care of the hemorrhaging risk.

Well-nourished mothers who eat good foods like green leafy vegetables and have adequate stores of vitamin K won't increase the vitamin K content of their breast milk even if they consume extra vitamin K foods or supplements.

Good sources of vitamin K: green leafy vegetables, Brussels sprouts, cabbage, milk, meat, eggs, cereal, fruit, and liver.

The regular use of antibiotics can kill the intestinal bacteria that help synthesize vitamin K. Since about half of the vitamin K we need is made within our digestive tracts, long-term use of antibiotics can deplete vitamin K stores. Talk to your doctor if you have taken or are taking a long-term course of antibiotics.

Vitamin C

Vitamin C helps form collagen, the substance that supports bones and teeth. It is an antioxidant, which means it protects other vital substances in the body from harmful chemical reactions. It also helps fight infection and assists with the absorption of iron.

While you're pregnant, the vitamin C concentration of your blood actually decreases. This probably occurs because your blood volume increases and your blood becomes more dilute. Your baby, on the other hand, has a vitamin C concentration in his blood twice that of yours.

The vitamin C content of breast milk can vary a bit depending on how many vitamin C–rich foods are eaten daily. Your baby consumes 24 to 40 milligrams of this important nutrient each day from your breast milk. You'll need to eat 95 milligrams of vitamin C daily in the first six months of lactation and 90 milligrams daily in the next six months to meet the needs of you and your baby.

Getting enough vitamin C for both of you is not hard to do

providing you make fruits, vegetables, or juices part of meals. If your intake of vitamin C is poor, breast-milk concentration will be maintained with vitamin C from your own body reserves. However, since body stores of vitamin C are minimal, you can't rely on them to meet your needs. Instead, make sure to eat vitamin C foods daily.

Recognizable vitamin C deficiency is rare today, but reports in older literature document a case of scurvy in a breastfed baby whose mother wasn't consuming enough vitamin C. The concentration of vitamin C in breast milk goes up a bit during the summer, when more fruits and vegetables are eaten. Supplements can increase concentrations of this nutrient in breast milk if the mother's diet has been deficient. Studies show that the vitamin C content of breast milk will level off at 50 to 60 milligrams per liter if a mother's intake meets or exceeds 100 milligrams daily.

Good sources of vitamin C: citrus fruits (oranges, grapefruits, tangerines, and so on), juices made from these fruits, fortified fruit juices, and most vegetables (dark green leafy vegetables, tomatoes, even potatoes and peppers).

Keep in mind that a real plus of getting enough vitamin C is that it enhances iron absorption. This is critical to your baby—and to you too, since many moms have low iron stores during pregnancy and lactation.

Thiamine (Vitamin B₁)

Thiamine is a member of the B vitamin family. It helps in energy production and the maintenance of a normal appetite and nervous system. Your need for thiamine increases to 1.6 milligrams while you're breastfeeding. Only about 0.13 to 0.21 milligrams of that will be consumed by your baby via breast milk. The thiamine requirement for a nursing mother is set quite a bit higher than what her baby consumes because thiamine plays a vital role in turning all the extra food and energy a mother consumes into breast milk.

Thiamine is not a hard nutrient to obtain, but wise food selections must be made. It is estimated by the National Academy of Sciences, Subcommittee on Nutrition During Lactation that a mother eating 1,800 or 2,200 calories a day will fall short of the recommended amount of thiamine. Fortunately, the RDA has a safety margin, and even though your thiamine intake might be a bit below the RDA, vitamin deficiency won't occur unless your diet is missing this nutrient for a very long time.

Low intakes of thiamine by mothers can result in lower thiamine concentrations in breast milk. In countries where mothers consume most of their calories from white rice that is not fortified with thiamine, breastfed babies have developed infantile beriberi, the disease caused by thiamine deficiency.

Good sources of thiamine: enriched bread or cereal, whole grain bread, cereal, and pasta, beans, nuts, meat, and liver.

Riboflavin

Riboflavin is another B vitamin. Like thiamine, it plays a role in energy production. It is also promotes good vision and healthy skin.

Your baby will consume 0.21 to 0.35 milligrams of riboflavin every day from your breast milk. To replace that and meet your own needs, the RDA is set at 1.8 milligrams in the first six months of lactation and 1.7 milligrams in the second six months. The RDA is set quite a bit higher than the amount the baby needs because mothers don't utilize riboflavin with 100 percent efficiency. The riboflavin content of breast milk seems to decline naturally with prolonged breastfeeding. This reflects the baby's need to start on solid foods himself so he can meet his own riboflavin needs.

Though there are no reported cases of riboflavin deficiencies in exclusively breastfed babies, mothers on low-calorie diets of

1,800 calories or less are at risk of not meeting their full RDA. Studies do show that riboflavin supplements can increase the content of this nutrient in breast milk even in mothers who eat an adequate diet. I have not come across any reports of excessive intakes or toxicity caused by riboflavin supplements, but it's still wise not to go overboard.

Good sources of riboflavin: milk, yogurt, cheese, whole grains, enriched bread and cereal, and green leafy vegetables.

Niacin

This water-soluble vitamin is found in food, but it can also be made in your body from the amino acid tryptophan. Niacin plays an integral role in our use and transfer of energy. It helps in the metabolism of sugar, fat, and alcohol and even works to keep our skin healthy.

While you were pregnant, your body became better at converting tryptophan to niacin, thereby guaranteeing you adequate supplies. A breastfeeding mom will secrete 0.9 to 1.5 milligrams of niacin in her milk each day. Milk from a well-nourished mother is adequate to meet her baby's needs. The RDA for nursing mothers is set at 20 milligrams of niacin. Even on a diet of only 1,800 calories a day, this level can be met if smart food choices are made. If for some reason you aren't able to eat enough niacin-rich foods, your body will convert tryptophan into niacin to meet your needs.

The niacin content of breast milk is directly affected by the food you eat, and niacin supplements can increase milk concentration. So choose supplements wisely.

Good sources of niacin: all protein foods (eggs, meat, poultry, fish, turkey, and tuna), whole-wheat bread, enriched pasta, cereal, bread, and nuts.

Vitamin B$_6$

Vitamin B$_6$ is extremely important for breastfeeding mothers. It assists in the proper metabolism of protein and fats and in the conversion of tryptophan to niacin. It also helps to make red blood cells.

Many mothers don't eat enough foods rich in vitamin B$_6$. You need 2.1 milligrams of this nutrient each day while breastfeeding; 0.06 to 0.09 milligrams will be secreted your breast milk. Many women eating low-calorie diets consume only 1.4 milligrams of vitamin B$_6$ daily. Some women who were long-term birth control pill users (4 to 12 years) before having a baby have had drastically low B$_6$ levels in breast milk. This is caused by the estrogen in the pills. Today's current "pill" has lower estrogen, but all new mothers should still eat lots of B$_6$-rich foods.

Don't take megadoses of vitamin B$_6$. Doses in the 300- to 600-milligram range have been observed to decrease milk production. Large doses of vitamin B$_6$ have been shown to cause neurological damage in women taking this nutrient for premenstrual syndrome. Select supplements cautiously if you use them. Doses of 2 to 6 milligrams do not appear to suppress milk production or cause dangerous side effects, but the National Academy of Sciences, Subcommittee on Nutrition During Lactation does not recommend the routine use of vitamin B$_6$ supplements for breastfeeding moms. It's best to meet your needs by selecting foods rich in vitamin B$_6$.

Good sources of vitamin B$_6$: meats, shellfish, chicken, turkey, eggs, beans, bananas, cauliflower, potatoes, whole grains, soybeans, and sunflower seeds.

Folic Acid

Folic acid, also known as folate and folacin, helps form hemoglobin in red blood cells and build new cells. Folic acid is frequently supplemented during pregnancy because the need for it is so great. A 1970 study even found that folic acid supplements reduced the incidence of premature births in its study group.

During pregnancy your folic acid requirement is set at 400 micrograms. For breastfeeding moms, the requirement drops to 280 micrograms. A day's supply of breast milk will contain about 50 to 83 micrograms of folic acid. (Human breast milk is a very good source of folic acid when compared to the milk of other animals. Goat's milk has only 10 micrograms per liter; half of the folic acid in cow's milk is destroyed when boiled or prepared for evaporated milk.)

Only about half of the folic acid you ingest gets absorbed, but the RDA is set high enough to allow for this inefficiency. A mother won't have much folic acid stored in her body because most excess folic acid is excreted in the urine. A mother can store about 6 milligrams of folic acid in her body, but after six months of exclusively breastfeeding, 12 milligrams will have been used. Simple math shows that a mother's reserves will be depleted unless she eats foods rich in folic acid. Foods must be selected carefully on a low-calorie diet: the average mother eating 1,800 calories per day will ingest only 261 micrograms, while a mother eating 2,200 calories will consume about 319 micrograms, more than the RDA of 280 micrograms.

Supplements can enhance the folic acid stores and the folic acid content of the breast milk of women deficient in this nutrient. Women with the folic acid deficiency called megaloblastic anemia will find that any dietary folic acid will go first to her breast milk to prevent the same anemia in her child. Women with healthy folic acid stores cannot enhance or boost the folic acid concentration of their milk with one-a-day supplements.

Good sources of folic acid: green leafy vegetables, beans, seeds, liver, eggs, and wheat germ.

Vitamin B_{12}

Vitamin B_{12} is a critical nutrient. It works with folic acid to build healthy red blood cells, and it also makes up part of the covering around nerve fibers. Vitamin B_{12} deficiency shows up as a creeping paralysis or a blood anemia characterized by large, immature red blood cells.

The RDA of vitamin B_{12} while you are breastfeeding is set at 2.6 micrograms; you'll be happy to know that this isn't hard to meet. It is estimated that even on as little as 1,800 calories a day, a mother will be able to ingest 5.2 micrograms. At 2,700 calories a day, that jumps to 7.8 micrograms.

It is thought that an infant needs about 0.3 to 0.5 micrograms daily, and studies show that mothers eating a good diet will secrete 0.6 to 1.0 micrograms each day in their breast milk. To reduce the risk of B_{12} deficiency even more, Mother Nature gives newborns a supply of vitamin B_{12} that can last as long as eight months—if their mothers have consumed enough B_{12} while they were pregnant.

A mother who eats animal foods such as beef, chicken, or dairy products can easily meet her vitamin B_{12} needs. Because fruits and vegetables are practically void of this essential nutrient, mothers who are strict vegetarians are at risk of B_{12} deficiency. A breastfed baby may show signs of the deficiency before his mother does.

To prevent B_{12} deficiency, pregnant and breastfeeding mothers who avoid all animal foods must take vitamin B_{12} supplements that provide the RDA. (If you are a vegetarian mother, read more about this in chapter 9.)

Good sources of vitamin B_{12}: any food of animal origin (beef, pork, lamb, turkey, chicken, fish, shellfish, milk, yogurt, cheese, eggs), soy milk, and breakfast cereal fortified with B_{12}.

Calcium

Calcium is the predominant mineral in bones and teeth, helping to build them and keep them strong. Calcium also helps muscles and nerves work properly, and it even plays a role in blood clotting and regulating blood pressure. Deficiency in childhood can show up as stunted bone growth; in adult women, the condition known as osteoporosis (weak, thin bones) has been linked with inadequate calcium intake.

While you are breastfeeding, your RDA is set at 1,200 milligrams daily—400 milligrams more than is needed by women who aren't pregnant. It can be very difficult if not impossible to meet this recommended intake if you aren't eating or drinking dairy products. Women on low-calorie diets (in the 1,800-calorie-per-day range) may be consuming only 715 milligrams, significantly less than the RDA.

Because this nutrient is so important, your body has some safety mechanisms that may go into effect if you don't eat enough calcium-rich foods. Studies have shown that women with chronically low calcium intake may be more efficient at utilizing the calcium they do eat. The RDA takes into account that your body is only 40 to 50 percent efficient at turning the calcium you eat as food into the calcium that will go into your breast milk.

At this point, you may be worrying that your calcium intake isn't good enough and your baby isn't getting enough of this vital nutrient. Rest easy. Once again, Mother Nature built in a safety mechanism to protect your baby. The calcium content of your breast milk will remain constant, but it will be done at your expense. If you don't eat enough calcium, your body will release calcium from your bones to make up the difference in your breast milk.

Because of this potential for increased calcium drain, there is concern that breastfeeding mothers might have an increased risk of osteoporosis. At this time there's not enough data to say how breastfeeding affects a woman's risk of osteoporosis. Some research suggests that breastfeeding itself may protect women from this disease.

If you are under age twenty-five, make sure you get lots of calcium. At this age, your bones still need to increase their strength by increasing their calcium content.

Black women have diets that average 30 percent lower in

calcium than those of white women. Low-income mothers also tend to have diets lower in calcium. Mothers who don't like or can't drink milk need to search out calcium-rich alternatives. (If you don't drink milk, read about what to do in chapter 9.)

The calcium in breast milk is more digestible than that found in cow's-milk formula. A breastfed baby will absorb two-thirds of the calcium in the breast milk he drinks. Formula-fed infants retain only about half of the calcium they consume. Formula-fed babies therefore need to ingest about 400 milligrams of calcium a day, while breastfed babies do just fine on the 168 to 280 milligrams they get in a day's supply of breast milk.

Good sources of calcium: milk, cheese, yogurt, fish with edible bones, tofu processed with calcium sulfate, bok choy, broccoli, kale, greens (collard, mustard, and turnip), and bread made with milk.

Phosphorus
Phosphorus is second only to calcium as the mineral in greatest quantity in your body. Most of it is found bound with calcium in bones and teeth. But it also makes up part of phospholipids (a type of fat) and is part of the buffer system that maintains the acid-base balance in your body. Phosphorus must also be present for your body to properly absorb calcium. The good news is that phosphorus is so abundant that deficiency isn't generally a problem.

Calcium and phosphorus are thought to be utilized best if they are present in equal amounts; therefore, the RDA for phosphorus is also 1,200 milligrams. The amount of phosphorus in your blood is very tightly regulated so that it stays at a constant level. What you eat, meal to meal, has very little impact on the phosphorus level of your breast milk.

Good sources of phosphorus: animal foods (all meats, fish, poultry, milk and dairy products) and soft drinks.

Excessive amounts of phosphorus can draw calcium out of your body to be excreted. Try to limit your intake of foods that are high in phosphates but low in calcium, including convenience foods processed with phosphates and soda.

Magnesium

Magnesium plays a necessary role in the release of energy. It also assists in proper muscle function and helps to keep calcium in teeth, which in turn helps prevent cavities.

If you eat lots of vegetables and whole grains, your diet is already rich in magnesium. Deficiencies aren't common except in illnesses associated with protracted vomiting or diarrhea, or in kidney disease. Scientists believe that a reservoir of magnesium is kept in our bones to prevent deficiencies.

About 21 to 35 milligrams of magnesium are secreted in breast milk daily, but your RDA is set at 355 milligrams, 75 milligrams more than when you weren't breastfeeding. The RDA is high because only half of the magnesium you eat is actually absorbed. Many mothers who don't eat vegetables and whole grains may just barely be meeting their magnesium needs.

Breastfeeding mothers consuming fewer than 2,200 calories a day will probably not be getting the recommended level of magnesium. On average, black women consume about 20 percent less magnesium in their diets than white women. This is because they select foods that contain less magnesium. Fortunately, the cases of magnesium deficiencies in breastfeeding moms are quite rare. Supplements of magnesium do not appear to increase magnesium concentration in breast milk.

Good sources of magnesium: nuts, seeds, legumes, whole grains, green vegetables, scallops, and oysters. Small amounts of magnesium are distributed in many foods, including spinach, tofu, sesame seeds, sunflower seeds, black-eyed peas, garbanzo beans, shrimp, beet greens, broccoli, navy beans, and lima beans.

Iron

Iron is a major part of the blood protein hemoglobin, which carries oxygen throughout your body. Women are particularly at risk for iron deficiencies because we lose iron every month during menstruation. Studies show that as many as 14 percent of women between the ages of fifteen and forty-four may have impaired iron status because of poor diet. During pregnancy, menstruation stops but demands on iron increase: the baby requires iron from you, the placenta also takes iron, and blood is lost during childbirth. Your need for iron is most critical in the second half of your pregnancy.

Breastfeeding itself uses very little iron—only about 0.15 to 0.3 milligrams per day. This is less than the amount of iron that would have been lost during menstruation. Since breastfeeding often delays the return of menstruation, your iron stores can have a chance to replenish themselves while you breastfeed if your diet is rich in iron. Since the demand for iron seems less critical while breastfeeding, the RDA is set at 15 milligrams, down from the 30 milligrams you needed while you were pregnant.

If your periods resume while you are still nursing, the demands on your iron reserves can be quite high. You'll have to make sure you eat lots of iron-rich foods. If your intake is poor, you, not your baby, will suffer from anemia.

Iron deficiency in children is a serious problem. Worldwide, 43 percent of children under age four are at risk of consuming iron-poor diets. In the United States, children between the ages of one and two are at the greatest risk of iron deficiency; they have used up the stores they were born with and now must rely on iron from food sources.

Breastfeeding is a superb way to get iron into your baby. It is estimated that half of the iron in human milk is absorbed by infants, while only 7 percent of the iron in formula is absorbed.

It is the lactoferrin, or "milk iron," in breast milk that helps your infant absorb iron and even helps her to fight intestinal infections.

Mothers who only partially breastfeed their babies will want to make sure that the other feedings, whether formula or introductory baby foods, are rich in iron. Two studies have found that babies still being exclusively breastfed at nine months are at greater risk for iron deficiency than babies eating some solids. This suggests that iron-rich foods should be introduced to all babies by the time they are six months old.

Your coffee drinking can also affect your baby's iron status. In Costa Rica, mothers drinking more than three cups of coffee a day while pregnant and breastfeeding had lower concentrations of iron in their breast milk, and their babies' iron status was affected by the time they were one month old. (Read more about coffee in chapter 8.) Iron absorption can be enhanced by eating a vitamin C–rich food with every meal. Don't, however, count on milk to help with iron; it is a very poor source of iron.

Good sources of iron: red meat, liver, fish, poultry, shellfish, eggs, beans, dried fruit, oysters, spinach, lima beans, dried peaches, navy beans, soybeans, and kidney beans.

Zinc
Zinc plays many vital roles, helping to maintain the good health of your eyes, liver, kidneys, muscles, skin, and reproductive organs.

The need for zinc is greater during the first six months of breastfeeding than at any other time in a woman's life. The RDA during this six months is 19 milligrams, which drops to 16 milligrams during the second six months of breastfeeding. Meeting this requirement is not easy to do, even for a woman consuming 2,700 calories a day. At lower calorie intakes, mothers may be getting only half or two-thirds of the RDA.

The RDA for zinc for breastfeeding mothers is set quite high, at least four to thirteen times the amount they will pass to their babies in milk (a mother will secrete about 0.9 to 1.5 milligrams of zinc daily in her breast milk in the first six months). The RDA is set so high because it is estimated that only 20 percent of the zinc we eat actually gets absorbed.

The good news is that low intakes by the mother are not generally reflected in a lower zinc concentration in her breast milk. Once again, however, your body may drain your own zinc reserves to provide for your baby if you don't consume enough of this important mineral.

Breast milk is rich in zinc, and colostrum is eight times richer in zinc than mature milk. The zinc found in breast milk is extremely absorbable. The zinc in formula is less so; formula must contain extra zinc to insure the baby gets enough.

In general, severe zinc deficiencies are not found in women in developed countries, but meeting the RDA of zinc can be difficult, particularly if you don't eat meat. The use of supplements has at best a small effect on breast milk, but for the mother not eating zinc-rich foods a zinc supplement may help maintain her zinc reserves. Recent studies suggest that an inadequate supply of zinc may be the cause of low vitamin A levels. Conversely, too much zinc can actually interfere with the absorption of copper.

Good sources of zinc: meat (beef, lamb, pork), poultry, seafood (oysters, crab, shrimp), eggs, seeds, legumes, yogurt, whole grains (zinc from whole grains may not be as well absorbed as that from other zinc sources), black-eyed peas, and wheat germ.

Iodine

You need only tiny amounts of this mineral, but without it your thyroid gland couldn't function. An iodine deficiency manifests itself as goiter, or enlarged thyroid gland. Iodine is part of the thyroid hormone that regulates body temperature and metabolism.

The RDA for iodine is set at 200 micrograms for breastfeeding women, and it requires almost no effort to meet this total. Iodine accumulates in direct proportion to the mother's diet. Breast milk generally contains about 178 micrograms in a liter, but one study found that iodine levels in human milk can be as high as 731 micrograms per liter. At that level, the nursing infant would be getting ten times his RDA. For this reason, mother's shouldn't take iodine supplements.

Good sources of iodine: iodized salt, seafood, plants, and animals that are fed plants.

Selenium

This trace mineral works with vitamin E to protect body compounds from damage. Selenium usually appears in breast milk at a concentration of 20 micrograms per liter. The RDA for breastfeeding mothers is 75 micrograms per day, up 20 micrograms from when not breastfeeding.

Increasing your intake of a nutrient usually does not boost the concentration of that nutrient in your breast milk. Selenium is an exception to this rule. The selenium content of food varies throughout the world. In Africa, mothers eating native foods, which are often low in selenium, had low selenium concentrations in their breast milk. A study of vegetarian mothers in California who eat local foods rich in selenium found that their breast milk had high concentrations of this mineral.

Mothers secrete about 12 to 20 micrograms of selenium in their breast milk each day, and their babies probably absorb 80 percent of that. As with many other nutrients, when you consume only about 1,800 calories a day, meeting the RDA of 75 micrograms of selenium can be tricky. Increase your intake to the 2,200-calorie range, and meeting your needs won't be so hard.

Good sources of selenium: seafood (including canned tuna), organ meats, and grains.

Biotin

Biotin is a B vitamin that has not yet been widely studied. We do know that it assists carbohydrates, proteins, and fats in getting their important jobs done. It is widely available in many foods, and biotin deficiency is extremely rare.

Because a lot is not known about this nutrient, a specific RDA for breastfeeding mothers has not been defined. An intake of 30 to 100 micrograms daily is thought to be adequate for everyone over eleven years old.

There has been some concern that raw egg whites can bind and render useless the biotin you eat from other foods. While it is true that raw egg whites can bind with biotin, studies show that you'd have to eat about two dozen egg whites to get that effect. In any event, eating raw egg whites or whole uncooked eggs is not recommended because raw eggs may contain salmonella and cause serious illness in the person who eats them.

Good sources of biotin: egg yolk, yeast, liver, kidney, milk; some biotin is available in all plant and animal foods.

Pantothenic Acid

Pantothenic acid is a B vitamin that plays a small but vital role in energy metabolism. Though a deficiency in this nutrient is rare, it would manifest itself as vomiting, fatigue, insomnia, and perhaps diarrhea. The nutrient is abundant in so many foods that it's almost impossible not to get enough of it—any fatigue or insomnia you experience while breastfeeding is almost certainly not caused by a lack of pantothenic acid.

Pantothenic acid does not have an RDA defined by age. Instead, a broad range of 4 to 7 milligrams daily is thought to be needed by all adults, including nursing mothers. There have been no reports of deficiencies in breastfeeding mothers.

Supplements can increase the content of pantothenic acid in breast milk. In one study, four mothers taking a pantothenic acid supplement of 1 milligram or more had significantly greater levels of pantothenic acid in their breast milk as compared to mothers who did not take supplements.

Good sources of pantothenic acid: meat, fish, poultry, whole grain cereals, and dried beans.

Copper

Copper helps make red blood cells, heals wounds, and forms part of the protective covering around nerves. Copper deficiency is quite rare. The safe and adequate intake for copper is set at 1.5 to 3.0 milligrams per day, which should meet the needs of breast-feeding moms.

Animal studies show that copper is easily absorbed from breast milk, and so far there have been no case reports of any copper deficiency in breastfed babies. Furthermore, there does not appear to be a direct relationship between the amount of copper a mother eats and the level of copper in her breast milk. The copper concentration of breast milk naturally declines over the first four months of breastfeeding, at which time it levels off. Full-term healthy babies are born with a good supply of stored copper, and this reserve helps ensure that they have adequate copper available.

Good sources of copper: grains, nuts, organ meats, and seeds.

Manganese

This trace element works with your body's enzymes to help your metabolism function efficiently. The average adult has a reserve of only 18 milligrams in her entire body. The estimated safe and adequate dietary intake for manganese is 2.5 to 5.0 milligrams daily. This nutrient is widely distributed in many foods, and deficiencies have never been reported in humans.

Good sources of manganese: nuts, whole grain breads, cereals, pasta, meat, eggs, chicken, milk, and garlic.

Fluoride

Fluoride builds stronger teeth and helps fight tooth decay. It also makes up part of your bones. Though it is present in the body in only small amounts, insuring an adequate supply can almost guarantee healthier bones and teeth. Whenever the natural concentration of fluoride in local water supplies falls short of the desired level, supplements in the form of tablets or bottled fluoridated water advised. In most cases your pediatrician can tell you if the local water supply contains fluoride.

Too much fluoride, which is a concern to some health advocates, can cause discoloring of the teeth. A day's supply of fluoridated water contains about 1 milligram of fluoride. The estimated safe and adequate dietary intake for fluoride is 1.5 to 4 milligrams a day. It is unlikely that toxic levels could be obtained through drinking water alone.

Breast milk contains about 16 micrograms of fluoride per liter. The fluoride level of mother's milk isn't easily increased by what a woman eats. In fact, when a large dose of fluoride (approximately three times the RDA) was given to one mother, it barely increased the fluoride concentration of her breast milk.

The question of when and how much to supplement fluoride for a breastfed baby concerns and puzzles doctors. In the April 25, 1990, issue of the *Journal of the American Medical Association*, Dr. John Greene of the University of California School of Dentistry addressed this issue in a response to a letter to the editor. Dr. Greene recommends that mothers and pediatricians follow the fluoridation guidelines set by the American Academy of Pediatrics, which state that infants should receive 0.25 milligrams of supplemental fluoride daily if their water supply contains less than 0.3 parts per million of fluoride.

There have been many sensational stories about fluoride causing disease instead of preventing it. If you have a concern about drinking fluoridated water or using fluoride supplements, put your mind at ease by doing some investigating. Contact the American Dental Association or the American Academy of Pediatrics or talk to your health-care provider and ask for information. Your local library will be a good resource too. In our community the fluoride content of our public water supply is low. In hopes of preventing cavities I have followed our pediatrician's recommendation and given both Sarah and Emily daily fluoride tablets.

Good sources of fluoride: drinking water (if naturally fluoridated), fluoride tablets, tea, and seafood.

Chromium

Chromium works with the hormone insulin to regulate your body's blood-sugar levels and to help release energy from glucose. A specific recommended intake of this trace element has not been established for breastfeeding mothers, because not enough is known about their chromium needs. Instead, an estimated safe and adequate daily range of 50 to 200 micrograms has been established for all healthy individuals, including children, mothers, and other adults. Human breast milk contains approximately 50 micrograms of chromium per liter.

Good sources of chromium: brewer's yeast, calf's liver, American cheese, wheat germ, meat, unrefined foods, fats, and vegetable oils.

Molybdenum

Molybdenum sounds like something Superman might be afraid of. In fact, it's a trace element that makes up part of some essential enzymes in your body. We seem to need it in only minute amounts. Deficiencies of this nutrient are unknown, presumably because the amount we need is so small and isn't hard to obtain from food.

The estimated safe and adequate dietary range is thought to

be 75 to 250 micrograms per day. Molybdenum can prevent copper utilization, and for this reason supplements are not recommended.

Good sources of molybdenum: seafood, meat, grains, and legumes.

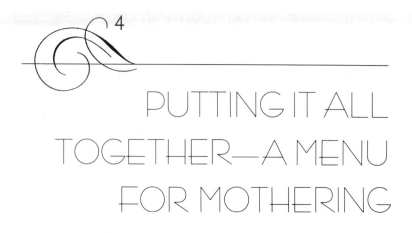

PUTTING IT ALL TOGETHER—A MENU FOR MOTHERING

HAVING CHARTS AND LISTS OF THE NUTRIENTS YOU NEED IS INteresting, but it doesn't necessarily help you decide what to eat for breakfast. In this chapter you'll see what a good, healthy menu entails and find some simple dos and don'ts that will keep you and your baby happy.

Nursing mothers can eat three meals a day plus three or four healthy snacks. You need more food while you breastfeed, and you'll feel better if you eat frequently.

WHAT SHOULD I EAT?

While you are breastfeeding you want to make sure you get enough of all the important nutrients. Let your own natural hunger pangs be of some help. Eat when you're hungry, but try to eat good, healthy food. A vegetable salad with whole-wheat bread on the side and some sliced chicken will provide you with many more nutrients than a Ring-Ding or Eskimo Pie.

There are certain foods you should try to eat every day (table 3).

Table 3. Outline of Your Daily Menu

A nursing mother needs to eat the number of servings shown from the six main food groups to meet her nutrient and calorie needs. The lists under each heading give you the serving sizes of various foods in that group.

Starch: 7–12 servings

Bread, 1 slice	Baked beans, ¼ cup
Bagel, ½	Beans (kidney, white, navy),
Pasta, ½ cup	⅓ cup, cooked
Cereal, ¾ cup	Rice, ½ cup

Protein: 7–8 ounces of beef, pork, lamb, veal, chicken, fish, turkey, or the equivalent. The foods below can be substituted for 1 ounce of meat.

Egg, 1	Canned salmon, ¼ cup
Tofu, 4 ounces	Oysters, 6 medium
Cottage cheese, ¼ cup	Peanut butter, 1 tablespoon
Dried beans, ½ cup cooked	

Milk: 3–4 servings

Milk, 1 cup	Yogurt, 8 ounces
Evaporated milk, ½ cup	Buttermilk, 1 cup
Tofu,* 1 cup	

Fruit: 3–6 servings. Choose at least one fruit rich in vitamin C (a citrus fruit is a good choice).

Apple, 1	Peach, 1
Cherries, 12	Papaya, 1
Pineapple, ¾ cup	Orange juice, ½ cup
Orange, 1	

Vegetables: 3–5 servings. A serving is ½ cup of any cooked vegetable or vegetable juice or 1 cup of any raw vegetable. Choose a dark green leafy or vitamin A–rich veggie daily.

Fat: 3–7 servings

Margarine or butter, 1 teaspoon

Mayonnaise, 1 teaspoon

Oil (corn, safflower, peanut), 1 teaspoon

Diet margarine, 1 tablespoon

Diet mayonnaise, 1 tablespoon

Cream, 1 tablespoon

*Tofu is not traditionally placed in the milk group, but it can be a good calcium source for mothers who don't drink milk. One cup of tofu at about 8 ounces contains approximately 308 milligrams of calcium, 172 calories, 18 grams of vegetable protein, and 13 milligrams of iron. One cup of milk contains 300 milligrams of calcium, 90 to 160 calories, 8 grams of animal protein, and 0.12 milligrams of iron.

If you eat the smaller number of recommended servings for all the food groups listed, select leaner meats, use 2-percent milk, and eat the portion sizes mentioned, the recommendations in table 3 add up to only 1,800 calories. A mother selecting the higher number of recommended servings will be eating about 2,700 calories a day. 2,700 calories is the intake recommended by the National Academy of Sciences. An intake of 1,800 calories is too low for most breastfeeding mothers—strive for a higher calorie intake.

HOW DO I KNOW IF MY DIET IS BALANCED?

To find out how well you are balancing your menu, write down everything you have to eat or drink for twenty-four hours. Include nighttime snacks and drinks. Review your twenty-four-hour menu and compare it to the food guide in table 3. Count foods only once; don't count cheese once in the milk group and once again in the meat group. Then answer these questions:

1. How many servings from the milk group did you
   have? _____
2. How many servings of meat, fish, chicken, cheese, or
   beans? _____
3. How many servings of fruit or fruit juices? _____
4. How many servings of vegetables? _____
5. How many servings of bread, cereal, rice, noodles, or other
   starches? _____
6. How many servings from the fat list? _____
7. How many "other" servings like soda, potato chips, cookies,
   jelly, candy? _____

Add up your groups and compare to the recommended number of servings. If you are far under or over on any of the food groups, you may be lacking in some vital nutrients. Try to balance your menu by adjusting your food choices to meet the suggested number of servings in all six categories.

Mothers who need to increase their calorie intake can choose the higher calorie selections within a group. For example, if a mom chose to eat a blueberry yogurt instead of milk, the calcium value would be almost the same but she'd eat 260 calories instead of the 120 in the low-fat milk. If she selected a half-cup of rice pilaf instead of an equal amount of plain rice, the calories would jump from 80 to 160.

Here are two different menus based on the six main food groups. They include all the recommended servings from every food group.

Menu One

Menu Two

Breakfast

Peanut butter on toast
Sliced banana with yogurt
Coffee or tea

Melted cheese on ½ bagel
Small bowl of cereal with
   milk and fresh fruit
Coffee or tea

Snack

Fruit and crackers	Fruited yogurt

Lunch

Chicken sandwich with lettuce, tomato, and mayonnaise Milk	Hamburger pizza, 3 slices Fruit juice

Snack

Pretzel sticks and cheese Water or herb tea	Angel cake with yogurt Water or herb tea

Supper

Baked fish Roasted potato with margarine Steamed carrots Salad with dressing Milk	Vegetarian lasagna (made with pasta, cheese, spinach, and tomato) Italian bread and margarine Poached pears

Snack

Yogurt topped with cereal and fresh fruit	Graham crackers and milk

The menus are quite different, but they both contain all the food groups mothers need. Portion sizes will determine the total calories and quantity of nutrients consumed. Mothers who want a more detailed guide to portions should read chapter 6.

CULTURAL DIFFERENCES

Not all mothers eat the same foods. Women of Asian or Hispanic heritage might select foods that are quite different from those on the menu of a woman of European background. Even though the foods are different, they can still be combined to provide a balanced, healthy menu. However, Hispanic or Asian-American mothers eating traditional diets may need to pay special attention to certain nutrients. Asian diets generally contain few dairy foods. A nursing mother eating a traditional Chinese or Asian diet will want to select foods such as tofu, bok choy, mustard greens, and calcium-fortified fruit juices to meet her calcium needs. One nutrition study found that Chinese-American adults did not consume enough folic acid, zinc, calcium, vitamins A and C, and iron to meet the recommended levels for these nutrients. Nursing mothers who eat traditional Chinese-American menus will want to make sure they get foods that contain these nutrients.

Young Mexican-American mothers eating traditional Mexican foods while breastfeeding have been found to have diets that are low in iron, vitamin A, and calcium. To boost calcium, mothers should be encouraged to eat low-fat cheeses and milk. Café con leche, a drink that is equal parts milk and coffee, can boost calcium, as can chocolate milk or hot chocolate. (Mothers don't want to drink more than two full cups of coffee a day because of its potential stimulating effect on their babies and because it might interfere with the mother's iron absorption.) Eating lean red meats will help boost iron. Red chilis in Mexican-style foods can be an excellent source of vitamin A.

MOTHERS SHOULD EAT THREE MEALS PLUS SNACKS

Eating frequently can actually help control hunger and overeating. Snacks that contain protein, complex carbohydrate, and some fat help keep your blood-sugar levels steady. If you skip meals or snacks, you may feel weak or famished. When you don't eat, your blood-sugar levels drop, signaling your hunger mechanism to make you want to eat. Sometimes you'll overconsume because you're so hungry.

Snacks that are rich in simple sugars like candy, sweetened fruit juice, or soda are rapidly digested. These foods give a boost to your blood sugar. Often, your body responds by overproducing insulin, the hormone responsible for keeping your blood sugar steady. When too much insulin is produced it can bring your blood sugar low enough to cause a new round of hunger. To prevent this cycle, simply eat regularly and eat foods like whole grains, fruits, vegetables, lean meats, and low-fat cheeses for snacks.

One word of warning about snacking. If you need to eat something at the 2:00 A.M. feeding because you're really hungry, then by all means have something to eat. But keep in mind that nighttime snacking can be a tough habit to break once you're no longer nursing and don't need the extra food.

DO I HAVE TO EAT BREAKFAST?

I think all breastfeeding mothers should eat in the morning. If you have gone all night without food, your body needs some refueling. Breakfast doesn't have to be bacon and eggs with a side order of hash browns. It can be much easier—and lower in fat.

Cereal is my favorite breakfast food because it's quick and nutritious. The added milk provides protein and calcium and the cereal itself is a rich source of B vitamins and zinc. Top it with fruit or drink a glass of juice and you've started yourself off on the right foot. (Unless you're eating a very large bowl of cereal —and some of us do—you'll probably need a side order of toast with it too.)

A good breakfast gives you about 25 percent of the energy and nutrition you need for the day, but I think it does even more. The habit of eating breakfast will serve you well long after you stop breastfeeding. Many people have more energy in the morning if they eat breakfast, and as we get older, breakfast seems to help in the fight against overeating and weight gain.

WHY DOES EATING BREAKFAST MAKE ME EVEN HUNGRIER?

I often hear this question from adults who are trying to control their weight. The answer may be that the taste of food after a nightlong fast triggers appetite. If no food had been eaten, that appetite might never have been stimulated. But this is no reason to skip breakfast. Instead, I recommend that you eat a healthy, low-fat morning meal and then have a snack later in the morning. After a week your body should adjust to the new routine and the hunger will dissipate. And remember, you should be hungry. You're the sole source of nourishment for your baby and you must eat enough for him, too. Listen to the signals your body is sending.

HOW MUCH WATER DO I NEED?

While you're breastfeeding you need to drink more fluids—at least two quarts every day. It doesn't have to be only water. Fruit juice, tea, and milk can all help to satisfy your need for fluids. Even fruits and vegetables contain small amounts of water.

A mother produces about 23 ounces of milk for her baby every day. You must replace those 23 ounces and take in extra fluid to meet your own body's needs. Water prevents dehydration, but it also helps to eliminate the body wastes created during metabolism. Water dilutes these wastes so that they can be excreted out of your body more easily.

It's frequently suggested that lots of extra water is needed to make breast milk and that if a mother needs to increase the volume of her milk she should drink more fluids. This is not true. Drinking more water does not make a mother produce more milk. Recently, nineteen healthy mothers and their babies participated in a study to measure the impact fluids have on breast-milk production. The nursing mothers in the study increased their fluid intake by over 30 percent, but there was no resulting increase in milk production.

Mothers who drink lots of water will urinate more often and have a lighter-color urine. Mothers who don't drink the recommended amounts will still produce an adequate supply of milk, but they will urinate less and probably complain of constant thirst.

Most mothers can rely on their thirst to tell them when they need more fluids. Drink as soon as you feel the first thirst sensations. One good way to get enough fluids is to take a drink of water every time you nurse your baby. Remember that when it is very hot, your need for liquids increases; make sure you drink a bit more in hot weather.

My sister Sheila gave me a great tip. Before you go to bed, fill a tall glass with ice cubes. Place it in the baby's room or wherever you nurse during the night. When the baby wakes for her nighttime feeding, the ice will have melted and you'll have a cold, refreshing glass of water to drink while the baby nurses.

WHAT FOODS SHOULD I AVOID?

Many mothers think they must survive on a bland diet while nursing. This isn't true. Mothers from many cultures breastfeed successfully on diets that are far different from ours. Feel free to use any seasonings you like. Using salt does not increase the sodium in your breast milk, and pepper won't make your milk spicy. Some foods do bother mothers; you can read more about this in chapter 8. The substances you do need to be careful with are alcohol and coffee. In general, limit coffee to two cups a day and alcohol to an occasional drink (more about this in chapter 8, too).

WHAT IS MOST IMPORTANT?

Don't focus on what you shouldn't eat. Instead emphasize all the good foods you *can* have. Calcium, zinc, magnesium, vitamin B_6, and folic acid are the nutrients you need the most. To get them, you'll want to eat whole grain cereals and grains, lots of green leafy vegetables, poultry, seafood, milk, cheese, yogurt, and lean cuts of meat. Not a bad way to lose weight, when you come to think of it!

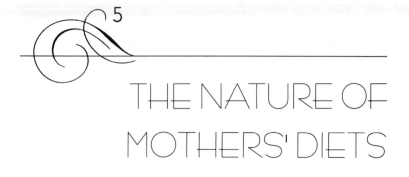

THE NATURE OF MOTHERS' DIETS

AT SOME POINT WHILE YOU'RE NURSING, YOU MAY BE INTERESTED in losing weight. Losing weight while you're breastfeeding is a completely different proposition than it was before you had your baby. This chapter will explain what to expect from your body as you lose weight and what is safe and what isn't.

HOW I GOT INTERESTED IN THIS SUBJECT

When I was pursuing my education in nutrition I was fortunate enough to have been accepted into an intensive thirteen-month training program at the Boston Lying-in Hospital, now known as the Brigham and Women's Hospital. The Boston Lying-in was a Harvard Medical School hospital that at the time delivered more babies than any other hospital in Boston. It was here that I first got to talk to new moms about their diets.

Our hospital was filled with women: some were in for surgery or tests, but most were new mothers. One of my regular assignments was to speak to every new breastfeeding mother about the role that good nutrition plays in a satisfying nursing experience. Of course, eight out of ten new mothers wanted to know how they could safely lose weight and still breastfeed their babies. No problem, I told them—one of the big extra bonuses of breastfeeding is that you can lose weight even while eating 2,700 calories a day.

In 1978, it was thought that nursing women could lose weight effortlessly because they needed so many calories to make milk and keep the baby well fed. This notion of automatic weight loss certainly seemed to make sense, and it was backed by the National Academy of Sciences.

Years later, a new study suggested that all mothers would probably not automatically lose weight if they ate the 2,700 calories being recommended for breastfeeding mothers. This study, published by Dr. Nancy Butte, found that breastfeeding mothers could successfully nurse their babies on far fewer calories than were usually recommended. I couldn't help but think that there were mothers all over Boston who were having trouble losing weight and would love to get their hands on that friendly dietitian trainee who told them to eat as much as they wanted.

CAN'T I JUST ENJOY BEING A MOM FOR A WHILE?

When I started writing this chapter, I had a conversation with my good friend Marta about weight loss. Marta has a four-year-old daughter, and our families have been friends since we met in a postpartum exercise class four years ago. "I think it's awful that mothers are pressured into losing weight while they breastfeed.

It's as if we're no good unless we're skinny. For goodness sake, we just had a baby and then we start to criticize ourselves for being overweight. Nobody bugs the fathers if they've put on a few pounds."

Marta's comments reflect the way a lot of mothers feel. There is tremendous pressure to be the "perfect" woman. Ads in magazines show skinny models who are on the edge of malnutrition. Ads on TV shows skinny new mothers who hold their tiny babies while they promote liquid diets. The not-so-subtle message is to strive for the media idea of perfection.

This book is not about being skinny and malnourished. It's about eating good food, enough to take care of you and your child. Don't do anything you don't feel good about. The last thing I want to do is add more pressure to a new mother's busy life. Raising and nursing a child is the most important job you can do.

If a breastfeeding mother wants to nurse and lose weight too, then the information in these chapters will help her meet her goals safely. If she doesn't want to lose weight, she can use the information to make sure she eats the foods that are essential to the good health of her and her child.

WOMEN, OBESITY, AND HEALTH

Approximately 25 percent of American women age thirty-five to fifty-five weigh 30 percent more than they should. Obesity is defined as 20 percent over ideal body weight. There are good reasons to pay attention to what you eat, and how much you weigh now. It's much easier to prevent a weight problem than to treat it later on. A recent study by Dr. Jo Ann Manson, published in the *New England Journal of Medicine,* found that of the 115,000 women she followed over an eight-year period, the ones who were heaviest had three times the risk of developing heart disease that the leanest women did. Obesity is also linked to other health problems like diabetes. Weight loss is not just about good looks. Your good health is at issue, too. A diet that keeps you in the range of your desirable weight* is also more likely to have a lower percentage of fat and contain lots of good, nutritious foods.

WHY LOSING WEIGHT WHILE BREASTFEEDING IS SO DIFFERENT

Giving birth and breastfeeding bring physical and emotional changes. Breastfeeding affects what you need to eat, and being a new mother reduces the time you have for cooking. Most new mothers complain of constant fatigue and an inability to accomplish anything: "I was home all day with the baby. I never put my feet up once, but I don't feel like I got anything done. You simply don't have the time or energy to follow complex dieting plans. In a study conducted at the University of California, Dr. Mary Wilson Blackburn asked twelve women to keep food and activity diaries while pregnant and while breastfeeding. The diaries revealed that once the mothers delivered their babies and were nursing, they spent 10 to 15 percent less time resting than they did while pregnant. The time lost to mom was spent on taking care of the new baby. So again, if you feel tired and don't have time to take care of yourself, you're not alone.

The good news is that proper nutrition can help prevent fatigue. Before becoming a mother, a woman might have been able to lose weight by skipping meals or just drinking liquids to cut calories. These strategies won't work now. If you curb your food intake too severely you won't get enough nutrition to maintain your health—and your baby's. A mother on a severely restricted diet can develop problems with her milk supply. Guess what happens? The mom has a fussy, hungry baby who requires even more care and probably makes her even more tired. To prevent exhaustion, you must eat enough to keep your energy

---

*See page 103 to find out how to calculate your ideal body weight.

reserves fueled. The trick is not to eat too much, and to eat the right foods.

Your need for nutrition is greater now than at any other time in your life. Perhaps when you lost weight before you cut down on breads, starches, or even dairy products. If you do that now, you may be restricting your intake of nutrients such as calcium and the B vitamins like thiamine. In most cases, if you don't eat enough of the essential nutrients, your body will automatically steal them from its own reserves, directing them to your breast milk so that your baby will be well nourished. This diversion of vitamins and minerals is fine if it happens only occasionally, but a continuous depletion of your own body stores could cause you health problems later on. Some researchers even believe that a mother's reserves may not always be adequate to compensate for her inadequate intake of nutrients.

The good news about breastfeeding is that you probably *can* eat more than you are normally accustomed to and still lose weight. Studies suggest that most of us won't be able to lose weight if we eat the full 2,700 calories recommended, but a woman eating 2,200 calories a day can lose weight. That 2,200 calories is a lot more satisfying than the 1,200 calories most women restrict themselves to when dieting.

GO SLOW

While you breastfeed, you should lose weight more slowly than you would otherwise. Safe weight loss for most adult women is thought to be one to two pounds per week, or about eight pounds a month. For breastfeeding moms, safe weight loss after the first postpartum month is thought to be only one to two pounds a month for the first four to six months, and not more than four and a half pounds a month.

For many of you, one to two pounds a month may sound painfully slow. But remember, you won't be depriving yourself, so you shouldn't feel hungry. If you nurse your baby for ten months, it could add up to a loss of ten to twenty pounds!

HOW THE WEIGHT COMES OFF

A European study reported that first-time mothers lost the most weight in the first few months after delivery. Older mothers with two or more children lost more weight between the third and sixth months postpartum. In an Australian study of 174 mothers, weight loss was found to level off by the sixth month.

Many women are unable to reach their prepregnancy weight until they stop nursing altogether. As long as you breastfeed, your breasts will add at least two to three pounds to the scale.

EXERCISE—IT'S DIFFERENT TOO

How much exercise and energy you use in a day changes considerably when you become a mother. Taking care of and feeding a child usually involves more housework and family chores, but this is rarely the kind of activity that burns calories. Many mothers find that being housebound with a new baby considerably curtails their activity levels. A small study of American women showed that sedentary breastfeeding moms used up only 1,800 to 1,900 calories in a day's activities (this did not include the calories they used to make breast milk). A comparison group of nonbreastfeeding mothers performing light to moderate activities burned up 2,200 calories.

This does not mean that all breastfeeding mothers burn fewer calories. If you are chasing around other busy toddlers or working in a strenuous job or even putting in a summer garden, your energy expenditure can be far greater than the 1,800 calories mentioned. In fact, in one study mothers exercising on a regular basis were able to expend 2,600 calories daily, and that did not include the approximately 500 calories used to make breast milk.

The bottom line is that while nursing you must be prudent about how you diet. There just isn't as much leeway in your nutritional needs. I'm a firm believer in taking it slowly. Lose weight by selecting food carefully; let the extra calories needed to breastfeed come from your own fat reserves. That way you burn fat while you eat nutritious foods and keep healthy.

POSTPREGNANCY WEIGHT LOSS

You're not alone if you expected to return to your prepregnancy weight once you delivered. Keep in mind that it took your body nine months to build your baby's first home. For many moms, it takes as long or longer to return to their prepregnancy size.

It can be helpful to understand where you kept the extra weight you carried while you were pregnant. If you had the textbook pregnancy and weren't overweight before you got pregnant, then you should have gained twenty-five to thirty-five pounds. If you were underweight before conception, your doctor may have encouraged you to gain twenty-eight to forty pounds or more. An overweight mom could have had a perfectly healthy baby and pregnancy with a weight gain of only fifteen to twenty-five pounds. Table 4 shows how those theoretical pounds would have been distributed.

Table 4. How Did I Gain So Much and Where Did It Go?

Infant at birth	5–10 pounds
Placenta	1 pound
Increase in mother's blood volume	4 pounds
Increase in mother's uterus and muscles	2½ pounds
Increase in breast tissue	3 pounds

Amniotic fluid that surrounds baby	2 pounds
Mother's fat stores	5–15 pounds
Total	22½ to 37½ pounds

Once your baby was born, there was obviously an immediate drop in weight caused by the delivery of the baby and the expulsion of the placenta. Since the baby was no longer relying on your blood supply, your own blood volume and fluid levels began to return to normal. You may have noticed you had to urinate more frequently while your body got rid of some unneeded fluid. Some women may temporarily retain fluid longer, and they may find that if they step on the scale they won't have lost as much weight as they expected.

There are no hard and fast rules about weight loss after birth, but one hour after delivery the average mother can expect to lose about thirteen and a half pounds. Between the first hour and twelfth day postpartum, another three and a half pounds should disappear. By the sixth week, any weight left above the prepregnancy level is fat and breast tissue.

HOW MUCH WEIGHT IS IT SAFE TO LOSE—AND HOW FAST?

Most breastfeeding mothers lose about one to two pounds per month over the first six months. This seems to be a normal and safe amount. A weight loss exceeding four and a half pounds per month is not recommended.

As I said before postpregnancy weight loss is unpredictable, with wide fluctuations from one mother to another. I was surprised that five days after the delivery of my eight-pound, twelve-ounce baby girl the scale showed I had lost only eleven pounds. Don't be too disappointed when your body doesn't instantly return to its prepregnancy shape. Don't be discouraged either if you must still wear maternity clothes to feel comfortable. Just take care of yourself—don't push weight loss now. In fact, don't even get serious about losing weight until at least six weeks after delivery.

WHAT IF I LOSE WEIGHT TOO FAST?

If you are losing weight too fast (more than four and a half pounds per month), then you really aren't eating all you should. Your total food intake isn't adequate, and therefore your intake of nutrients probably isn't adequate either. Inadequate intake of calories can diminish the amount of milk you produce, and rapid weight loss may cause the release of toxins stored in your body fat. (Read more about toxins and pesticides in chapter 8.)

WHAT DO I NEED TO BE CAREFUL ABOUT?

The risk associated with an overzealous and too-restrictive weight loss plan is that you may compromise your milk supply. In a study of short-term calorie restriction of breastfeeding mothers, Margaret Strode and coworkers at the Department of Pediatrics, University of California at Davis, discovered that when a small group of nursing mothers restricted their daily intake of calories from an average of 2,300 to about 1,600, there was no immediate change in their babies' weight gain or feeding schedule. In the week that followed the calorie restriction, however, there was a measurable difference. The babies did not take in as much milk, they fed less, and their rate of weight gain decreased. While mothers who strictly limit their calorie intake might see no immediate effect on their milk production, there may be repercussions in the days that follow.

Short-term fasting does not seem to harm milk production.

Two studies of mothers fasting from fourteen and a half to twenty hours found that there was no difference in milk secretion. This might be important for mothers who must fast for a short while for a medical test or for religious reasons.

CAN I USE LIQUID DRINKS OR DIET PILLS WHILE NURSING?

Liquid diets and weight loss medications are not recommended for nursing mothers. Many of the over-the-counter appetite suppressants control hunger with massive amounts of caffeine. If you use these products you can transfer the caffeine to your baby, possibly making him irritable and fussy.

In the May 1991 issue of *American Baby* magazine, Gail Kaitschuck, L.D., R.D., tells the story of a new mother who used an over-the-counter high-protein drink to lose the extra forty pounds she gained while pregnant. She started the liquid diet two weeks postpartum, while nursing her baby. Three weeks later she and the baby were hospitalized: the baby for failure to thrive because of inadequate milk supply and the mother for fatigue and low blood pressure. Both baby and mother were harmed because the liquid protein drink didn't meet the energy requirements for a breastfeeding mother. The liquid protein diets are simply inadequate and inappropriate for any breastfeeding mother.

WHEN SHOULD I START A DIET?

The Subcommittee on Nutrition During Lactation suggests that mothers not start weight loss diets until at least two to three weeks after they give birth, since curtailing calories any earlier might be detrimental to the nursing experience. The first few weeks of breastfeeding are important to establishing an adequate milk supply and to ensuring a good bond between you and your baby. I think new mothers should take at least six weeks before taking on any new challenges, including dieting.

IS IT NORMAL TO LOSE WEIGHT WHILE BREASTFEEDING?

Yes, most mothers lose one or two pounds per month while breastfeeding. A mother who is overweight should be able to lose up to one and a quarter pounds a week without adversely affecting her milk production. But not all nursing women will automatically lose weight.

When I reviewed the research about weight loss and breastfeeding I found several cases in which weight loss was quite slow or even nonexistent. In 1989, Dr. Marie Brewer reported the results of a study of the weight loss patterns of fifty-six new mothers. Twenty-one were exclusively breastfeeding, fifteen were exclusively formula feeding, and twenty were breastfeeding and using formula. The women's weights and measurements were taken within the first two days after they gave birth, then again at three and six months postpartum. There was no significant difference in the rate of weight loss between any of the groups of mothers. Those with lower pregnancy weights were likely to have greater weight loss. The mothers feeding formula to their babies ate a lot fewer calories than the breastfeeding mothers, but very few of the nursing mothers ate the recommended 2,700 calories a day, either.

In another study of twenty-seven well-nourished breastfeeding mothers conducted by Carolyn Manning-Dalton at the University of Connecticut, the women were weighed twelve days after giving birth. They weighed, on average, thirteen pounds above their prepregnancy weight. Over a subsequent three months, these mothers averaged a weight loss of approximately four and a half pounds while eating about 2,200 calories a day. The authors of this study concluded that breastfeeding does not automatically promote weight loss, and they suggest that the recommended 2,700 calories a day is more than most nursing mothers need.

At the First European Congress on Obesity held in 1988, a study of 1,423 women followed for one year postpartum was presented. The strongest predictor for weight retention was how much mothers gained while pregnant; women who gained more than the recommended amount had a harder time getting it off. Older mothers also retained more weight than younger moms. There were large variations in weight gains and losses, but the bottom line was that breastfeeding alone does not guarantee weight loss.

It has also been reported that women can actually gain weight while nursing. Of course, if a mother is below ideal body weight, weight gain is fine, but it could be a problem if she is overweight.

What can you expect? You'll probably lose some weight while you breastfeed, but you may not automatically shed all of the weight you put on while you were pregnant. Good food choices can help you lose those last pounds steadily without compromising your health or your nursing experience.

HOW MANY CALORIES DO NEW MOMS REALLY NEED?

A healthy mother who gained the recommended amount of weight while pregnant is believed to need an additional 500 calories per day while she nurses her baby. Mothers who weren't able to gain enough weight while pregnant may need 650 additional calories. Add these numbers to the 2,200 calories believed necessary for all women age fifteen to fifty and the total is 2,700 to 2,850 calories a day while you are breastfeeding. (Before the most recent RDA figures were published in 1989, the caloric need of nonpregnant women was set at 2,100 calories and breastfeeding mothers were said to need 2,600 calories daily.) The figure of 500 extra calories per day for all nursing mothers was calculated by the Food and Nutrition Board, a division of the National Academy of Sciences Institute of Medicine. It is estimated that the average mother makes about 750 milliliters of breast milk every day. It takes an additional 640 calories to make this milk. Approximately 100 to 150 of these calories are expected to come from the fat that you stored while you were pregnant. That leaves 500 calories you need to supply from food. Women who did not eat enough extra food to meet the requirement of 2,700 to 2,850 calories per day were thought to be at risk of jeopardizing their own health and possibly compromising their ability to breastfeed their babies.

Though these calculations look good on paper, they may not hold true for all of us when we actually try to plan out calorie levels that allow for good nutrition and reasonable weight loss. In fact, recent research suggests that if some of us were to follow these recommendations we might still be carrying around our pregnancy fat at our baby's first birthday.

In 1984, Dr. Nancy Butte, an expert on nutrition and lactation at the Children's Nutrition Research Center at Baylor College of Medicine in Texas, published a study that changed the way we think about calories during breastfeeding. She found that mothers were able to nurse their babies successfully and lose weight while consuming less than the 2,600 calories a day then specified in the RDA.

Dr. Butte studied the diets of forty-five breastfeeding mothers over a period of four months. These women were able to successfully nurse their babies while eating an average of only 2,186 calories. They were also able to lose an average of eleven pounds in the four months of the study. The 2,186 calories is more than 500 calories below the current RDA for breastfeeding mothers.

There are three possible reasons Dr. Butte's study came up with a different calorie level than the RDA. First, not all women produce the theoretical 750 milliliters of milk a day. In this study, the women produced only 735 milliliters, or 25 ounces, of milk. Second, breast milk is thought to contain 67 to 77 calories per 100 milliliters. In Dr. Butte's study, it averaged only 64 calories per 100 milliliters. Finally, the base level of 2,200 calories needed each day by nonpregnant women may be too high to begin with.

Another factor influencing caloric needs is that nursing mothers may use calories more efficiently. Dr. P. J. Illingworth studied nineteen healthy new mothers. Twelve were breastfeeding and seven were bottle feeding. Seven nonpregnant nonlactating women participated as controls. The study, published in a 1986 issue of the *British Medical Journal,* examined how breastfeeding mothers utilize calories. He found that breastfeeding enhances a woman's metabolic efficiency and that new mothers may not need to increase their calorie intake to the level that is currently recommended.

As you can see, deciding how many calories you need while breastfeeding isn't simple. The current recommendation for mothers who want to breastfeed is 2,700 calories per day; at the very least, mothers are advised to eat 1,800 calories a day. This recommendation was suggested by the Subcommittee on Nutrition During Lactation and published in *Nutrition During Lactation* in 1991. The 2,700-calorie level probably guarantees an adequate diet, assuming the mother makes reasonable food choices. But as the research studies suggest, 2,700 calories may be too much for some mothers and may cause weight gain or prevent weight loss.

Don't automatically assume you should cut down to the 1,800-calorie level. Mothers eating only 1,800 calories a day must pay very close attention to getting adequate supplies of calcium, zinc, magnesium, vitamin B_6, and folic acid. It is important for mothers to realize that when calories are restricted, food is restricted and nutrients may be harder to get. This is the time you need to be well nourished, so plan menus carefully. Because the research and data on what breastfeeding mothers really need to eat isn't entirely clear, don't rely completely on what the doctors or scientists recommend. Instead, listen to your own body. Eat enough so that you feel good and your baby is happy, but don't feel compelled to stuff yourself. The next chapter will help you make the healthful food choices that will be best for you and your baby.

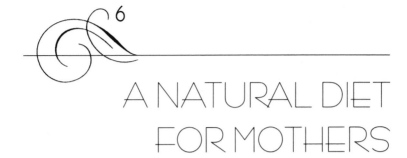

A NATURAL DIET FOR MOTHERS

Your goal while breastfeeding is to eat enough food to keep healthy and satisfied. On the pages that follow I'll give you enough information to let you eat well, lose weight gently, and have a happy nursing experience.

Normally, when planning diets and menus, clients are asked to weigh and measure the food they cook and eat. This kind of precision is often needed to manage disease. But breastfeeding mothers aren't sick. As a result, you have much more flexibility in your food choices and portions, as long as you eat enough to meet your increased need for calories and to get the nutrients such as vitamin B_6, calcium, and zinc that your body craves.

The dietary system I use incorporates nine food groups. Use the food groups and suggested menus that follow to make decisions about what to eat and to guide you in planning healthy meals. You should eat well but allow your body to do what it is supposed to do: use up the fat you stored while pregnant. Just as breastfeeding is the natural continuation of pregnancy, gentle weight loss can be the natural course of events while breastfeeding.

WILL I BE ON A DIET?

I don't like the word "diet" because it sounds as if you'll have to change your eating habits just long enough to reach the dress size you envision. Once you reach that weight goal, you'll feel you can indulge in all the "forbidden" foods again. That's not the way to ensure healthy, permanent weight loss. Please don't think of this as a "diet" if that means a short-term change. Instead, think of it as a time to take stock of your eating habits and make some permanent changes for the better.

HOW MUCH CAN I EAT?

My Natural Diet for Mothers is like no other diet you've been on. Instead of being based on deprivation, this menu is meant to meet your calorie needs and satisfy your appetite. In fact, you may feel like you have never eaten so much food before. You're probably right.

Remember that, on average, mothers secrete 420 to 700 calories each day in their breast milk, and that it takes even more calories to make that milk. Without even increasing your activity, your body will be needing many more calories than you are probably accustomed to. Also, the foods that I recommend are packed with nutrition but low in fat and empty calories. I might recommend that you eat the equivalent of three slices of bread, three ounces of protein, a serving of fruit and vegetables, and a cup of yogurt for lunch. These foods are rich in the B vitamins, calcium, and folic acid that mothers need, but they add up to only 500 calories. A quarter-pound hamburger with cheese, french fries, and a Coke would give you close to 1,000 calories without being as rich in some important nutrients.

As far as I'm concerned, there isn't a single food you can't have, no matter how rich in calories, fat, or sugar. (The only exception would be foods or drinks high in alcohol or caffeine.) It's not the one candy bar or the occasional piece of birthday cake that gets you into trouble. It's your whole pattern of eating that counts.

WHERE DO I START?

Begin by reading the one-day sample menu. It supplies about 2,700 calories, plus all the nutrients you need. The food is distributed in three meals and three snacks. The 2,700 calories is based on the recommendations of the Food and Nutrition Board of the National Academy of Sciences Institute of Medicine, which determines the recommended dietary allowances for nutrients and calories.

The 2,700-calorie total was determined by adding the 2,200 calories needed each day by women age fifteen to fifty to the 500 extra calories required to make breast milk, for a total of 2,700 calories. (In the first six months, mothers are thought to expend, on average, 640 calories to make a day's supply of breast milk. The allowance for calories is set at only 500 because it is expected that mothers can draw on the fat stores they gained while pregnant to make up any needed calories.) As I explained in chapter 5, these calculations may not be accurate for some mothers, because those mothers may need less than the baseline 2,200 calories. A more individualized plan can be developed, as I'll show you later, but the 2,700-calorie menu is a good place for most mothers to start.

HOW DO I USE THE NATURAL DIET FOR MOTHERS?

Follow the meal plan and menu guide in this chapter to make smart eating choices. If you need to modify the caloric content, just follow the adaptation guidelines I give in the discussions of the individual food groups.

A NATURAL DIET FOR MOTHERS

At no other time in your life will you be likely to eat 2,700 calories a day and still expect to lose weight. Your goal is to get the 2,700 calories but to do it in a way that meets your needs for nutrition. To meet that caloric need in a balanced diet you'll want to eat the following number of servings daily from the six main food groups:

Nonfat milk—4
Protein—8
Vegetables—5
Fruit—6
Starch—12
Fat—7

These six categories are the key to a healthy diet. My system adds three other groups as well: free group, combination group, and the daily option group of foods to eat only once a day. The free, combination and daily option foods add flavor and variety to your meals, but they aren't nutrition powerhouses.

These food groupings are based on a menu-planning system called Exchange Lists for Meal Planning.* This system is used

---

*This material has been modified from Exchange Lists for Meal Planning, which is the basis of a meal planning system designed by a committee of the American Dietetic Association and the American Diabetes Association. While primarily designed for people with diabetes and others who must follow

by many dietitians and nutritionists. The foods in any given group are similar to one another in nutrient and calorie content and can therefore be swapped freely for one another.

In order for a food to be placed in a category it must be similar in the amount of calories, carbohydrate, protein, and fat to the other foods in the group. Portions are designed so that every food in a group will have the same number of calories per serving. For example, one slice of bread has approximately 80 calories, as does one-half bagel. These two foods from the starch group can be substituted for each other without increasing or decreasing the calories in a meal.

The food groups can appear a bit confusing at first, but read through them, work with them a bit, and you'll find they are extremely useful. Using these nine food groups, a mother might come up with the following menu for a day's meals. This menu gives her the recommended amounts of calories and nutrients, provides plenty to eat, and tastes good, too.

One Day's Sample Menu

Food group	*Amount*	*Sample Food*
Breakfast		
Milk	1	1 cup nonfat milk
Protein	1	1 egg, poached
Fruit	2	1 cup orange juice
Starch	3	3 slices toast
Fat	2	2 teaspoons margarine
Free	–	Coffee/tea
10:00 A.M. Snack		
Milk	½	½ cup yogurt
Starch	1	¾ cup corn flakes
Fruit	1	½ banana, sliced

special diets, the exchange lists are based on principles of good nutrition that apply to everyone (© 1989 American Diabetes Association, The American Dietetic Association).

Lunch

Milk	1	1 cup milk
Protein	3	3 ounces sliced chicken
Starch	2	1 roll
Vegetable	2	1 tomato, sliced, and 1 cup salad
Fat	3	2 teaspoons mayonnaise and 1 tablespoon salad dressing

2:00 P.M. Snack

Protein	1	1 tablespoon peanut butter
Starch	1	3 graham crackers
Fruit	2	1 cup grapefruit juice
Vegetable	1	1 cup vegetable sticks

Supper

Milk	1	1 cup nonfat milk
Protein	3	3 ounces cooked steak
Vegetable	2	½ cup carrots, ½ cup green beans
Starch	4	2 cups noodles
Fat	2	2 teaspoons margarine
Fruit	1	1 peach

9:00 P.M. Snack

Milk	½	½ cup milk
Starch	1	¾ cup cereal

LEARNING TO USE THE EXCHANGE SYSTEM

Because foods in the lists are grouped by their caloric and nutritional profiles you might be surprised where some of them turn up. For instance, cheese is in the meat group because it contains protein and has a similar calorie content as meat foods. Corn and potatoes are very rich in carbohydrate, so they find their niche in the starch group, not the vegetable group. A food like pizza will be found in the combination food group since it is made up of starch (crust), protein (cheese), and fat (oil). If vegetables top that pizza, then a serving from the vegetable group would be added too.

My meal plans use nonfat milk. Nonfat milk has the same calcium value as whole cow's milk, but the fat and calorie content is quite a bit lower. I encourage mothers to think of nonfat milk as the preferred choice and whole milk as nonfat milk with an extra 1½ pats of butter. If you really are stuck on whole milk you can have it, but you should use less of the foods allowed in the fat group, such as butter or margarine. You'll notice that I list margarine instead of butter in my menus. That is because margarine is made from vegetable oils and contains no cholesterol. Both margarine and butter have the same calories. If you love butter and do not have a cholesterol problem, then feel free to use it as your fat serving. Just stick to the portion sizes I recommend.

You don't want to trade from different food groups. If you don't eat all your fruit servings, that doesn't mean you can eat extra from another food group, because the calorie and nutritional composition would be different. If you do mix and match food groups, you might not get the balance you strive for.

CAN I EAT THE SAME FOODS MY FAMILY EATS?

Absolutely. The same meals, fruits, vegetables, rice, bread, and so on that other family members eat should be part of your diet, too. The only foods a breastfeeding mother should avoid are those with lots of caffeine or alcohol. Because a mother's calorie needs increase while she's nursing, even the occasional fried food is allowed. What is most important is that you get enough of the six main food groups to supply you with the nutrition you need.

THE NINE FOOD GROUPS

On the following pages is a detailed list of all the foods within each group. At the beginning of each food group read about the specific nutrition those foods provide. Pay close attention to the minimum number of servings suggested.

Both a minimum and a recommended daily serving are listed with each food group. The recommended daily serving numbers equal a 2,700-calorie balanced menu. The minimum servings add up to only 1,800 calories a day. A breastfeeding mother who does not eat the minimum recommended number of servings from the various groups may not be able to meet all her nutritional needs.

The recommended minimum daily number of servings from each food group is:

Food Group	Recommended Minimum Servings
Milk	3
Protein	7
Fruit	4 (1 vitamin C rich)
Vegetable	4 (1 dark green leafy or vitamin A–rich)
Starch	7
Fat	5
Free foods	No recommended amount
Combination foods	No recommended amount
Daily option foods	1 (optional)

Starch Group

These foods are rich in carbohydrate and low in fat. They are also good sources of thiamine, niacin, and iron. Whole grain foods will be good sources of fiber, and bran cereals are good sources of zinc. Each serving will give you roughly 80 calories, 15 grams of carbohydrate, 3 grams of protein, and a trace of fat.

Recommended daily amount	12 servings
Minimum daily amount	7 servings

Food	Serving Size
Bread (white, rye, raisin, whole wheat, pumpernickel)	1 slice
Bagel, English muffin, pita bread; hamburger, hot dog, or sandwich roll	½
Tortilla	1
Cereal (flake type, unsweetened)	¾ cup
Cereal (Grape-Nuts, wheat germ, bran concentrate)	⅓ cup
Cereal (uncooked oatmeal or farina)	½ cup
Grains—rice (brown, white, instant), bulgur, grits, pasta, noodles	½ cup uncooked
Beans and peas (lentils, kidney, split, black-eyed, lima)	⅓ cup uncooked
Corn	½ cup or 1 ear
Potato (white, sweet)	½ cup mashed or 1 small
Winter squash (acorn, butternut)	½ small
Crackers/snacks	
Breadsticks	2 4-inch sticks
Animal crackers	8

Food	Serving Size
Graham crackers	2
Popcorn	3 cups
Crisp crackers (melba toast, pretzels, Ry-Krisp, saltine, nonfat whole wheat)	3–6
Angel cake	1½-inch slice
Gingersnaps	3
Sherbet	¼ cup
Frozen yogurt	⅓ cup

The following are starchy foods that also contain about 5 grams of fat. Eating one serving of these is like eating a starch and a fat; in other words, a slice of bread with butter on it. If you choose these foods, try to cut back on the number of fat servings you eat at the meal.

Popover, scone, donut, biscuit, corn bread, muffin, waffle, pancake, coffee cake	1 small serving
Chow mein noodles or fried rice	½ cup
Crackers with fat added	4–6
Taco shells	2
French fries	10
Homefries	½ cup
Cupcake (unfrosted)	1
Plain cake (unfrosted)	1 small serving
Cookie	1 3-inch round
Granola-type cereal	¼ cup

Milk Group

The foods listed below provide approximately 90 calories, 12 grams of carbohydrate, 8 grams of protein, and just a trace of fat per serving. They are also a rich source of vitamin D, riboflavin, and calcium. Nonfat and low-fat milks are encouraged over whole milk because they are equal in nutrition but have many fewer fat calories.

Recommended daily amount   4 servings
Minimum daily amount   3 servings

Food	Serving Size
Nonfat, ½-percent, 1-percent milk	1 cup
Dry nonfat milk	⅓ cup
Evaporated nonfat milk	½ cup
Low-fat buttermilk	1 cup
Plain, nonfat yogurt	1 cup

Not all mothers drink the milks listed above, so the following foods can be used as additional sources of calcium. Note how the calorie, protein, and fat composition of these foods differ.

Food	Calories	Carbo-hydrate (g)	Protein (g)	Fat (g)	Calcium (g)
Skim milk, 1 cup	90	12	8	trace	300
Tofu, 8 ounces	172	6	18	10	308
Collards,* 1 cup cooked	51	9.5	5	1	299
Kale, 1½ cups cooked	65	10	8	2	310
Turnip greens, 1 cup cooked	29	5	3	0.3	267
Beet greens,* 2 cups cooked	52	10	5	0.6	288
Spinach,* 2 cups cooked	82	13	11	1	330

*These vegetables may contain significant amounts of oxalic acid, which can interfere with calcium absorption. For this reason, don't rely on them as your only calcium source.

Food	Calories	Carbo-hydrate (g)	Protein (g)	Fat (g)	Calcium (g)
Fruit yogurt, 1 cup	225	42	9	3	314
Goat's milk, 1 cup	168	11	9	10	326
Kefir, 1 cup	160	9	9	5	350
Chocolate milk, 1 percent, 1 cup	160	26	8	3	287
Soy milk,** 1 cup	79	4	7	5	10

**Soy milk might look and taste similar to milk, but it is extremely low in calcium.

Protein Group

One serving of each food listed below will contain approximately 7 grams of protein, 3 to 5 grams of fat, and 55 to 75 calories. These protein foods are also good sources of iron, zinc, and thiamine.

Recommended daily amount	8 servings
Minimum daily amount	7 servings

Food   Serving Size

Food	Serving Size
Meat (beef, veal, pork, venison, rabbit, liver, organ meats, poultry without skin, fish)	1 ounce
Canned fish in water (tuna, salmon, crab)	¼ cup

Food	Serving Size
Oysters	6
Cottage cheese, ricotta cheese	¼ cup
Parmesan cheese	2 tablespoons
Mozzarella, low-fat cheeses	1 ounce
Lunch meats, low calorie	1 ounce
Egg	1
Egg substitute	¼ cup
Tofu	4 ounces
Beans (great northern, navy, kidney, lima, black-eyed peas)	½ cup cooked
Beans baked with pork and sweeteners	½ cup *

*Baked beans contain about 8 grams of protein in a ½-cup portion, but the 175 calories per portion is significantly higher than the 75 calories per serving for other foods in this list.

These protein foods are higher in fat and calories. Try to use them less frequently.

Cheese, regular	1 ounce
Sausage	1 ounce
Cold cuts	1 ounce
Hot dog	1
Nut butters	1 tablespoon

Vegetable Group

The foods in this group provide approximately 25 calories per serving. They also contain 5 grams of carbohydrate, 2 grams of protein, and are a good source of vitamin A and vitamin C as well as fiber. Choose a dark green leafy or orange vegetable three or four times a week.

Recommended daily amount	5 servings
Minimum daily amount	4 servings

A serving is ½ cup cooked vegetable or juice or 1 cup raw vegetable

Food

Asparagus	Mushrooms
Bean sprouts	Okra
Beans, green and wax	Onions
Beets	Pea pods
Broccoli	Peppers, all colors
Brussels sprouts	Rutabaga
Cabbage	Sauerkraut
Carrot juice	Spinach
Carrots	Tomatoes
Cauliflower	Tomato juice
Eggplant	Turnips
Greens	Yellow squash
Kohlrabi	Zucchini
Leeks	

Starchy vegetables such as peas, corn, and potatoes are listed under the starch group.

Fruit Group

Each serving provides approximately 60 calories and 15 grams of carbohydrate. These foods are a rich source of fiber and vitamin C.

Recommended daily amount	6 servings
Minimum daily amount	4 servings

Food	Serving Size
Apple, kiwi, nectarine, orange, peach, pear	1 whole
Plums, persimmons, tangerines, apricots, figs	2 small
Berries	1 cup
Melon cubes	1 cup
Juice (apple, grapefruit, orange, pineapple)	½ cup
Juice (cranberry, grape, prune, cherry)	⅓ cup
Applesauce, fruit cocktail	½ cup
Banana	½ large or 1 small
Cherries	12
Grapes	15
Mango	¾ cup or ½
Papaya	1 cup or ½
Pineapple, canned	⅓ cup
Pomegranate	½
Dried fruit	
Apples	4 rings
Apricots	7 halves
Dates	2
Figs	2
Prunes	3
Raisins	2 tablespoons

Fat Group

These foods contain approximately 5 grams of fat per serving and 45 calories. Foods that come from animal sources contain cholesterol.

Recommended daily amount	7 servings
Minimum daily amount	5 servings

Food	Serving Size
Margarine, mayonnaise, all cooking oils, butter	1 teaspoon
Diet margarine, diet mayonnaise, mayonnaise-type salad dressing	1 tablespoon
Salad dressing, oil variety	1 tablespoon
Diet salad dressing	2 tablespoons
Olives	10 small, 5 large
Nuts	
Peanuts	10 large, 20 small
Cashews, pine nuts, sunflower seeds	1 tablespoon
Almonds, dry roasted	6
Cream	
Heavy	1 tablespoon
Light	2 tablespoons
Sour	2 tablespoons
Cream Cheese	1 tablespoon
Coffee whitener, liquid	2 tablespoons
Coffee whitener, powder	1 tablespoon
Gravy, homemade or canned	1 tablespoon

Free Foods Group

These foods are so low in calories that they don't need to be considered in your total food intake, but in most cases they don't have much nutritional value either. Sugar-free products are listed here, but I rarely encourage the use of sugar substitutes or the products that have them. I only recommend them if a person has diabetes. All breastfeeding mothers can afford the 10 to 20 calories in a teaspoon of sugar, honey, or jam—so enjoy the real thing.

Food

Bouillon
Carbonated drinks, diet
Carbonated water and club soda with fruit flavors
Cocoa powder, unsweetened
Coffee or tea (Limit all coffee to 2 cups a day, black tea to 2 to
   3 cups. Herb tea is caffeine free and can be enjoyed in
   reasonable quantities)
Drink mixes, sugar free
Tonic water, sugar free
Nonstick pan spray
Fruit
   Cranberries, raw
   Rhubarb, raw
Vegetables
   Celery
   Chinese cabbage
   Cucumbers
   Green onions
   Hot peppers
   Radishes
Salad greens
   Endive
   Escarole
   Lettuce
   Romaine
Candy, hard, sugar free
Gelatin, sugar free
Gum, sugar free
Jam or jelly, sugar free
Sugar substitutes such as saccharin or aspartame
Whipped topping, 2 tablespoons
Condiments
   Catsup

Food

Horseradish
Mustard
Pickles, dill, unsweetened
Taco sauce
Vinegar
Seasonings
Dry or fresh herbs and spices
Flavoring extracts (almond, butter, lemon, peppermint, vanilla, walnut, etc.)
Hot pepper sauce
Lemon
Lemon juice
Lime
Lime juice
Soy sauce
Wine used in cooking
Worcestershire sauce

Combination Food Group

Much of the food we eat is mixed together in various combinations that don't fit easily into only one food group. It can be quite hard to tell what is in a certain casserole or baked food. The list below gives you average exchange values for some typical combination foods.

Food	Exchange Value
Meat and cheese casseroles, made with noodles, rice, or potato, 1 cup	2 starch, 2 protein, 1 fat
Cheese pizza, 2 small slices	2 starch, 1 protein, 1 fat
Chili with beans, 1 cup	2 starch, 2 meat, 2 fat
Chow mein without noodles or rice, 2 cups	1 starch, 2 vegetable, 2 protein

Food	Exchange Value
Macaroni and cheese, 1 cup	2 starch, 1 protein, 2 fat
Soups	
Bean, 1 cup	1 starch, 1 vegetable, 1 protein
Chunky, all varieties, 1 10¾-ounce can	1 starch, 1 vegetable, 1 protein
Cream, canned, made with water, 1 cup	1 starch, 1 fat
Vegetable, without potatoes or corn, 1 cup	1 vegetable
Vegetable, with potatoes or corn, 1 cup	1 starch
Sugar-free pudding made with nonfat milk, ½ cup	1 starch

Daily Option Group

These foods don't really fit into any category, but they taste good and a nursing mother can certainly enjoy them. They provide calories but very little nutrition. Try to use only one of these foods a day. One serving provides about 50 calories. The sugar-free alternatives can be used, but since I don't encourage the use of artificial sweeteners (unless a mother is diabetic), I'd rather see you enjoy the real thing.

Food	Serving Size
Maple syrup	1 tablespoon
Jam or jelly	1 tablespoon
Life Savers	6 pieces
Regular soda	6 ounces
White or brown sugar	1 tablespoon
Honey	1 tablespoon
Chocolate candy	½ ounce
Chocolate syrup	1 tablespoon

ONE WEEK'S MENU

The following seven-day menu has been computer analyzed for nutritional content, provides about 2,700 calories, and meets 100 percent of the nutrient needs of breastfeeding mothers. You can follow this sample exactly or use the food exchanges given as a good reference for designing your own menu. It's best if you follow a menu for a whole day; this way, you'll get a truly balanced diet. If you wish, you can also mix and match breakfasts, lunches, and suppers from different days. The balance might not be as perfect, but no harm will be done. Water, coffee, and tea are free foods, and you can include them at any meal (but first, read about coffee in chapter 8). Recipes for foods marked with an asterisk are included in chapter 10.

A Week's Menu for Breastfeeding Mothers

DAY ONE

Food	Exchanges
Breakfast	
1 cup fruit juice	2 fruit
¾ cup bran flakes	1 starch
1 cup skim milk	1 milk
1 English muffin with 2 teaspoons margarine	2 starch, 2 fat
Snack	
½ cup plain yogurt with 1 tablespoon honey or syrup	½ milk, 1 daily option
6 graham crackers	2 starch
Lunch	
Quick-Cooking Chili,* 1¾-cup portion	3 protein, 2 starch, 2 vegetable, 1 fat
1 cup salad with 1 tablespoon dressing	1 vegetable, 1 fat
1 cup skim milk	1 milk

Snack

1 slice cheese melted on ½ pita bread with chopped tomato	1 protein, 1 starch, 1 vegetable
½ cup fruit juice	1 fruit

Supper

4 ounces salmon, broiled	4 protein
1 cup skim milk	1 milk
1 cup steamed carrots with 1 teaspoon margarine	2 vegetable, 1 fat
1 baked potato	1 starch
1 cup salad with 1 tablespoon dressing	1 vegetable, 1 fat
1 small ear of corn with 1 teaspoon margarine	1 starch, 1 fat
Small bunch of grapes	1 fruit

Snack

½ cup skim milk	½ milk
1½ cups cereal	2 starch
½ banana	1 fruit

DAY TWO

Food	Exchanges

Breakfast

Two-egg vegetable omelet (Melt 1 teaspoon margarine in omelet pan, add 2 beaten eggs. Let set a bit. Sprinkle with ½ cup of mixed vegetables; try tomato, mushroom, and onion. Cook until done.)	2 protein, 1 fat, 1 vegetable
1 English muffin with 1 teaspoon margarine	2 starch, 1 fat
1 cup orange juice	2 fruit

Snack

Yogurt shake (1 cup plain yogurt blended with 1 cup strawberries)	1 milk, 1 fruit
2 slices raisin toast with 1 teaspoon margarine	2 starch, 1 fat

Lunch

Crab salad sandwich (3 ounces crabmeat, canned or fresh, 1 tablespoon diet mayonnaise, and chopped celery or onion on a whole-wheat roll)	2 starch, 3 protein, 1 fat
1 cup Broccoli Salad*	2 vegetable, 1 fat
1 cup skim milk	1 milk

Snack

½ banana	1 fruit
2 rice cakes	1 starch
½ cup skim milk	½ milk

Supper

4 ounces Vegetable Meat Loaf*	4 protein, 1 vegetable, 1 starch
2 small oven-roasted potatoes	2 starch
½ cup green beans with 1 teaspoon margarine	1 vegetable, 1 fat
1¼ cups strawberries	1 fruit
1 cup skim milk	1 milk

Snack

1 bagel with 1 tablespoon cream cheese	2 starch, 1 fat
½ cup skim milk	½ milk

DAY THREE

Food	Exchanges

Breakfast

½ grapefruit	1 fruit
1 cup yogurt with 3 tablespoons wheat germ and 10 sliced grapes	1 milk, 1 starch, 1 fruit
2 slices toast with 2 teaspoons margarine	2 starch, 2 fat

Snack

½ cup skim milk	½ milk
1 tablespoon peanut butter on 1 slice toast	1 protein, 1 starch

Lunch

Tuna sandwich (½ cup tuna with 2 teaspoons mayonnaise on 2 slices toast with sliced tomato)	2 protein, 2 fat, 2 starch, 1 vegetable
1 cup carrot and cucumber sticks with diet dressing	1 vegetable, 1 fat
1 cup skim milk	1 milk
1 apple	1 fruit

Snack

¼ cup cottage cheese on 1 bagel with sliced tomato	1 protein, 2 starch, 1 vegetable
1 cup fruit juice	2 fruit

Supper

3 Salmon Croquettes*	4 protein, 1 starch, 1 fat
½ cup Yogurt Dill Sauce*	½ milk
1 cup steamed carrots	2 vegetable
1 cup cooked rice with 1 teaspoon margarine	2 starch, 1 fat
Baked Pear*	1 fruit, 1 daily option
½ cup skim milk	½ milk

Snack

½ cup skim milk	½ milk
3 cups salted air-popped popcorn	1 starch

DAY FOUR

Food   Exchanges

Breakfast

3 slices French toast (3 slices whole-wheat bread dipped in 2 eggs scrambled with ½ cup milk. Cook in 1–2 teaspoons of margarine until done. Sprinkle with nutmeg.)	3 starch, 2 protein, ½ milk, 1–2 fat
Top with ½ cup yogurt and 1 cup Blueberry Sauce*	½ milk, 1 fruit, 1 daily option
½ cup orange juice	1 fruit

Snack

3 graham crackers	1 starch
¾ cup skim milk	¾ milk

Lunch

1 cup vegetable soup	1 vegetable
1 pita filled with Curried Chicken*	3 protein, 1 fat, ¼ milk, 1 fruit, 2 starch
1 cup Broccoli Salad*	2 vegetable, 1 fat

Snack

3 graham crackers	1 starch
1 cup fruit juice	2 fruit

Supper

1 cup skim milk	1 milk
3 ounces marinated steak	3 meat
1 cup mashed potato with 1 tablespoon gravy	2 starch, 1 fat
½ cup corn kernels with 1 tablespoon margarine	1 starch, 1 fat

1 cup green beans with 1 teaspoon margarine	2 vegetables, 1 fat
1 slice angel cake with strawberries	1 starch, 1 fruit

Snack

½ cup skim milk	½ milk
8 animal crackers	1 starch

DAY FIVE

Food	Exchanges

Breakfast

1 cup skim milk	1 milk
1½ cups bran flakes with ½ banana, sliced	2 starch, 1 fruit
1 slice toast with 1 tablespoon peanut butter	1 starch, 1 protein
1 cup orange juice	2 fruit

Snack

½ cup skim milk	½ milk
3 graham crackers	1 starch

Lunch

Mexican salad sandwich (Sauté 2 ounces ground turkey in 1 teaspoon vegetable oil and ¼ cup salsa. Divide between two warmed soft flour tortillas. Top with 1 ounce grated cheese, sliced lettuce, and tomato.)	3 protein, 2 starch, 1–2 vegetable, 1 fat
1 cup skim milk	1 milk
1 apple	1 fruit

Snack

½ cup apple juice	1 fruit
½ bagel with 1 tablespoon cream cheese	1 starch, 1 fat
½ cup milk	½ milk

Supper

2 pieces Yogurt-Fried Chicken*	4 protein, ½ milk, 1 starch
1 cup cooked carrots and green beans with 2 teaspoons margarine	2 vegetable, 2 fat
1 cup salad with 1 tablespoon dressing and 1 tablespoon sunflower seeds	1 vegetable, 2 fat
1 cup cooked rice with 1 teaspoon margarine	2 starch, 1 fat
⅓ cantaloupe	1 fruit

Snack

½ cup skim milk	½ milk
4 breadsticks	2 starch

DAY SIX

Food	Exchanges

Breakfast

2 slices raisin toast with 2 teaspoons margarine	2 starch, 2 fat
1 cup yogurt with ½ cup fruit and 3 tablespoons wheat germ	1 milk, 1 fruit, 1 starch
1 cup orange juice	2 fruit
1 ounce sausage	1 protein

Snack

½ cup yogurt with 3 tablespoons wheat germ and 1 tablespoon honey	½ milk, 1 starch, 1 daily option
½ banana	1 fruit

Lunch

Brown Rice and Broccoli*	2 starch, 3 protein, 2 vegetable, 1 fat
1 orange	1 fruit
1 cup skim milk	1 milk

Snack

1 hard-cooked egg with 2 teaspoons mayonnaise on 2 slices toast with sliced tomato	1 protein, 2 fat, 2 starch, 1 vegetable

Supper

3 ounces roast turkey	3 protein
1 cup stuffing with 1 tablespoon gravy	2 starch, 1 fat
1 cup steamed broccoli and carrots with 1 teaspoon margarine	2 vegetable, 1 fat
¼ cup sherbet with ½ cup sliced peaches	1 starch, 1 fruit
1 cup skim milk	1 milk

Snack

½ cup skim milk	½ milk
3 graham crackers	1 starch

DAY SEVEN

Food   Exchange

Breakfast

1 English muffin with 2 teaspoons margarine	2 starch, 2 fat
1 cup skim milk with ¾ cup cereal	1 milk, 1 starch
½ banana	1 fruit
1 cup orange juice	2 fruit

Snack

½ cup skim milk	½ milk
3 gingersnaps	1 starch

Lunch

3 ounces lean cold cuts on a roll with 2 teaspoons mayonnaise	3 protein, 2 starch, 2 fat
1 cup skim milk	1 milk
1 cup sliced tomato and cucumber salad with 1 tablespoon French dressing	1 vegetable, 1 fat

Snack

1 ounce sliced cheese on ½ cup apple or pear slices	1 protein, 1 fruit
⅔ cup frozen yogurt	2 starch

Supper

1 cup skim milk	1 milk
1 cup Quick Spaghetti Sauce* over 1½ cups pasta	4 protein, 1 vegetable, 3 starch
1 cup salad with 2 tablespoons diet dressing	1 vegetable, 1 fat
1 cup cooked zucchini with 1 teaspoon margarine	2 vegetable, 1 fat
½ cup apple juice	1 fruit

Snack

Fruit frappé (½ cup plain yogurt blended with ¼ cup sherbet or frozen yogurt and ½ banana or 1 cup strawberries)	½ milk, 1 starch, 1 fruit

CAN I SNACK AT NIGHT?

Many mothers look forward to a special snack once the children are put to bed. This is a time to put your feet up, have an undisturbed conversation, or just savor the taste of a yogurt sundae in peace. I don't want to take this pleasure away from you, but I do suggest that you select something that is healthy and low in fat. Any of the snacks listed in the seven-day menu would do.

WHAT IF I DON'T EAT THE FOODS ON THE MENU?

Menu plans can't match the likes and dislikes of everyone who uses them. That's the beauty of the food-exchange system. If I recommend three starches at breakfast, it doesn't matter if you eat three slices of toast or one and a half bagels or a cup and a half of oatmeal. All three foods are similar in nutritional value and calories. You can choose the food you like. What I don't recommend is switching from one food group to another, eating fewer servings, or skipping meals or snacks altogether.

YOUR MENU LASTS FOR ONLY ONE WEEK—WHAT DO I DO AFTER THAT?

Use this menu as a guide. It's meant to be enlightening, not enslaving, so please don't feel you must be ruled by it. It can help you learn about how much food you need and which foods will help provide the nutrients you need. Even if you plan to follow my menu exactly, you'll soon find that rigidity won't always work. Special occasions do come up; a friend drops by with sub sandwiches and your menu says crabmeat salad. Or maybe your mother baby-sits for an evening so you can treat yourself to a much-deserved dinner out. Try to be flexible.

HOW WILL I KNOW IF I'M GETTING ENOUGH TO EAT?

If you're hungry all the time or are losing more than one pound per week, you're probably not eating enough. The best way I know to evaluate your food intake is to keep a food diary. Write down what you eat and the exchanges the foods represent, and compare your list to the servings I have recommended from each food group. If you aren't eating the minimum number of servings from any of the groups, you must start eating more. If you have no appetite and can't seem to make yourself eat, talk to your doctor or find a registered dietitian for personalized advice.

I FEEL AS IF I NEED TO EAT MORE AT THE MORNING SNACK— WHAT SHOULD I DO?

Once again, don't be a slave to my menu. It's fine for you to switch the portions around, but try not to go below or above the recommended number of servings from any food group. If you want to add fruit to your morning snack, add it and consider skipping the fruit suggested for the afternoon snack.

WHAT IF THE 2,700-CALORIE MENU ISN'T RIGHT FOR ME?

The 2,700-calorie menu may not be right for some women. Mothers who resume running or other active sports may actually need many more calories. Women who find motherhood brought an abrupt halt to their exercise routine may need quite a bit fewer calories. And after six months of nursing, when your baby starts on more and more solid foods, he'll no longer be relying on you as his sole source of nourishment, and you may not need to make as much milk or eat as many calories. If you still need to lose fat and your weight loss has stopped, you'll also need to modify the 2,700-calorie menu.

HOW TO INDIVIDUALIZE YOUR MENU

If you don't lose weight while eating 2,700 calories a day, you may need to eat fewer calories. Don't just stop eating or skip meals. Instead, use the worksheet in table 5 to determine your calorie needs more precisely. Using this information, you'll be able to adapt the Natural Diet for Mothers to help you lose weight. But remember, never go below the daily minimum number of servings of any food group while breastfeeding.

Table 5. Estimating Your Calorie Requirements

First, determine your goal weight (also called ideal body weight, or IBW):

Medium frame	Allow 100 pounds for the first 5 feet of height plus 5 pounds for each additional inch
Small frame	Subtract 10 percent from total for medium frame.
Large frame	Add 10 percent to total for medium frame.

For example, a medium-frame 5′8″ woman should weigh 140 pounds.
   Your goal weight or IBW is _____.

   Then multiply your goal weight by the activity number that matches your exercise habits. Most of us fall in the sedentary category unless we engage in regular exercise. Mothers who exercise 20 to 30 minutes three times a week are engaging in moderate exercise. If you are doing less exercise, count yourself in the sedentary group. If you exercise more often and for a longer duration, then you are probably engaging in heavy exercise.

13 for   Sedentary activity
(Some walking, typing, sewing, ironing, cooking, seated and standing activities, light housekeeping)

15 for   Moderate activity
(Walking briskly, weeding, hoeing, carrying loads, bicycling, tennis, dancing)

20 for   Heavy activity
(Jogging, heavy manual labor, climbing, digging)

Your daily calorie requirement when not breastfeeding is (IBW × activity number) _____.

Finally, add the 500 calories needed each day to make breast milk to this total.

Your daily calorie requirement when breastfeeding is _____.

For example, if your goal weight is 140 pounds and you are usually sedentary, you'd multiply your activity number of 13 by 140 pounds and come up with 1,820 calories. This is the number of calories you'd need if you weren't breastfeeding and wanted to maintain your ideal weight. Since you are breastfeeding, you need to add 500 calories, for a daily total of 2,320 (round it off to 2,300).

Those 2,300 calories should allow adequate nourishment for you plus just enough to ensure an adequate supply of breast milk while encouraging your body to burn some of the fat you stored while pregnant.

WHAT IF I WAS UNDERWEIGHT WHEN I DELIVERED MY BABY?

If you didn't gain enough weight while pregnant, you'll want to eat an extra 650 calories a day instead of 500 while you breast-feed. This amount should keep you from losing any more weight. To gain weight you may need to eat even more, perhaps a total of 3,000 calories per day.

CALORIES AREN'T THE WHOLE STORY

Calories are important, but there's more to losing weight safely. After all, a mother could eat 2,300 calories of ice cream every day and lose weight, but she'd feel miserable because her intake of essential nutrients would be inadequate.

Use your calorie needs as the starting point for planning a good, healthy diet. Nutritionists now recommend that we break up our calorie intake as follows:

Protein = 20 percent of total calories or a bit less
Carbohydrate = 50 percent of total calories or up to 60 percent
Fat = 30 percent of total calories or less

These percentages will affect your food choices differently at different calorie levels (table 6). Round your expected daily calorie level off to the nearest hundred and find how many servings of each food group you should choose each day.

Table 6. Food Choices for a Balanced Menu

Daily Calories	Milk (skim)	Meat	Starch	Vegetable	Fruit	Fat
1,800	3	7	7	4	4	5
1,900	3	7	8	4	4	5
2,000	3	7	9	4	4	6
2,100	3	7	9	4	5	6
2,200	3	7	10	4	5	7
2,300	3	7	10	4	6	7
2,400	4	8	10	4	6	7
2,500	4	8	11	4	6	7
2,600	4	8	11	5	6	7
2,700	4	8	12	5	6	7
2,800	4	9	12	6	6	8
2,900	4	9	13	6	6	9
3,000	4	9	13	7	6	10

Servings is a spanning header across the Milk, Meat, Starch, Vegetable, Fruit, and Fat columns.

Caution: At under 2,300 calories a day, your intake of calcium may be low because you're only getting three milk servings. To insure adequate calcium, choose at least one good alternate vegetable calcium source, such as a healthy serving of green leafy vegetables, or choose cheese, tofu, or canned fish with bones as one of your protein selections.

At 2,200 calories and below mothers must make very good food selections to meet all their nutrient needs. They may have a difficult time getting calcium, zinc, vitamin B_6, folic acid, magnesium, thiamine, iron, selenium, vitamin E, riboflavin, and niacin. Mothers eating near or at the 1,800-calorie level will need a multivitamin (read about supplements in chapter 2).

To adjust the week's menu to meet the calorie level you have calculated for yourself, simply compare the servings listed for your new calorie level to those for the 2,700-calorie diet and adjust accordingly. For example, a mother needing 2,500 calories a day would eat one less starch serving and one less serving from the vegetable group.

HOW OFTEN SHOULD I CHECK MY WEIGHT?

Check it only if you feel the need to and no more than once a week, preferably first thing in the morning on the same day of each week. (Try not to let the scale be your only guide to good health. I recommend that you focus attention on eating good food and getting regular, gentle exercise. If you are able to combine these two, then the scale will start to head in the direction you want.

CAN I HAVE SUGAR?

Sugar contains about 15 calories per teaspoon. It provides no nutrition, but if used in small amounts, I don't believe it does any harm. Personally, I prefer the taste of honey as a sweetener, but neither honey nor sugar can be called nutritious.

Honey and sugar are part of my daily option group. One serving of these foods a day is fine.

DOES A WOMAN WITH A BIGGER BABY NEED TO EAT MORE FOOD THAN I DO?

Babies need to eat about 45 calories a day per pound, so a baby weighing three pounds more than yours needs an extra 135 calories a day. If both babies are exclusively breastfed, the bigger baby will need to get that extra food from her mom's breast milk, and her mother will need to eat more than you to provide it. If the larger baby is more than six months old, she can get her extra calories from eating solids (preferably iron-rich foods) instead of from her mom.

SHOULD I EAT LESS WHEN MY BABY STARTS TO EAT SOLIDS?

By the time she's six months old, a baby can start on solid foods. In fact, a baby *should* start on solids then because she needs the nutrients, such as iron, that supplemental foods provide. There is no exact way to determine your calorie needs when your baby is nursing and eating solids. I suggest you let your appetite and body weight guide you. If you aren't hungry between meals, then you're probably getting all the food you need. If you're losing more than one pound a week, then you probably need to eat more. If you have reached your ideal weight, you want to eat enough to prevent further weight loss.

I DON'T WANT TO LOSE ANY MORE WEIGHT BUT I CAN'T STOP!

Some women can't keep weight on while breastfeeding. Frequent snacking and three good sit-down meals can help. You should also keep a food record and evaluate whether you're getting all the servings you need from the recommended food groups. If not, add the ones you're missing. If you are getting the amounts you thought you needed but you're still losing, then add an extra 200 calories per day by adding two starches and one extra serving of lean meat, or an extra cup of low-fat milk and one starch serving.

WHAT IF I NEED MORE HELP WITH MY DIET?

Nothing beats sitting down with a registered dietitian or a lactation consultant who has training in nutrition for personal guidance. But you can do a good job of evaluating your own diet by keeping a food diary. If you don't have time, a checklist like the one shown in table 7 can do just as well. Each time you eat a food, check off the food group it belongs in. Use one check for each serving you consume.

Table 7. Food Checklist

Each time you eat, check off the food groups consumed, one check for each food-exchange portion. For example, if you eat two slices of toast with two teaspoons of margarine at 7:00 A.M., you should place two checks in the starch box and two in the fat box in the 6:00 A.M. to 10:00 A.M. time slot. If you eat a combination food, check all the food groups that make up the dish. For example, 1½ cups of a casserole may merit two checks in the starch group, one in the protein, and one in the fat category. Free foods don't need to be marked, but put one check at the bottom of the page for each daily option food consumed.

Exchange Portions Eaten

6:00 A.M.–10:00 A.M.

Protein _____

Starch _____

Milk _____

Fruit _____

Vegetable _____

Fat _____

10:00 A.M.–2:00 P.M.

Protein _____

Starch _____

Milk _____

Fruit _____

Vegetable _____

Fat _____

2:00 P.M.–6:00 P.M.

Protein _____

Starch _____

Milk _____

Fruit _____

Vegetable _____

Fat _____

6:00 P.M.–10:00 P.M.

Protein _____

Starch _____

Milk _____

Fruit _____

Vegetable _____

Fat _____

10:00 P.M.–6:00 A.M.

Protein _____

Starch _____

Milk _____

Fruit _____

Vegetable _____

Fat _____

Daily Option _____

Now add up the checks in each category, enter them below, and compare your actual intake of each food group with the servings recommended in table 6:

	Actual intake	Recommended intake
Protein	_____	_____
Starch	_____	_____
Milk	_____	_____
Fruit	_____	_____
Vegetable	_____	_____
Fat	_____	_____

THE KEY TO YOUR SUCCESS IS STARTING OVER

In my experience, the greatest obstacle to weight loss and improved eating is that we think dieting is an all or nothing proposition. We start off highly motivated, but when we stray and eat what we think is inappropriate or "bad," we give up. It's very important to understand that you will never be a "perfect" eater. There will be times when all goes right and other times when you overeat or eat a high calorie–high fat food. The key to dietary success is to just start over. So please don't be disappointed in yourself if you don't eat the perfect menu every meal and every day. Just reestablish your goals and start over as often as you need to.

EXERCISE—
IT'S WORTH IT

ADDING EXERCISE TO YOUR INCREDIBLY BUSY LIFE MAY SEEM IM-
possible (or masochistic) but it's worth doing. A new mother
can get some much-needed toning from exercise, along with a
wonderful sense of well-being. After all, you take care of the
baby, but who's taking care of you?

The benefits of exercise are numerous. It maintains good muscle tone and protects against back pain. A sound exercise program can help prevent heart disease, osteoporosis, and obesity.
It even helps with depression. Exercise does more than just burn
calories; it actually increases your metabolism. One study found
that after a person exercises, her metabolic rate (the speed at
which she burns calories) can increase by 10 percent, and it can
stay that way for up to forty-eight hours. And instead of making
us hungry, exercise usually acts as an appetite controller.

*It doesn't really matter what you do. The key to an exercise program
is to find something you like and just do it.*

WHEN CAN I START TO EXERCISE?

Only your doctor knows the answer to this since he or she knows your medical condition. If you had an uncomplicated delivery and are in good health, you can probably start right away. A mother who had a caesarean birth may need to wait four weeks or more.

A woman who has recently given birth is in a unique physical state: she suddenly stops balancing the weight of her pregnant abdomen at the same time as she undergoes musculoskeletal changes that can leave her a bit unsteady. Add this to the fact that most of us aren't active in those last months of pregnancy, and you can see why you need to take it slowly at first. You have a lot of demands on you, and there's no need to overdo it.

BABIES CAN CHANGE OLD EXERCISE HABITS

Once your bundle of joy arrives, finding time for exercise can be much more difficult. If you arrange to have a half hour of time to call your own, you may have to choose between going for a walk, doing the laundry, or taking a much-desired nap.

Before I had children, I could schedule a walk anytime I felt like it. As a result I had no schedule, and at the end of the week my plans for taking three full walks had resulted in only one actual walk. After having Sarah, it was terribly difficult to arrange time for myself. The only way to pull it off was to schedule an appointment with my husband so that he could take care of her. Now we have two little girls and we still have to schedule regular exercise periods. I now get more exercise than I ever did in my life, and so does David.

Be realistic about what you can take on while caring for a new baby. It's great if you can manage to have fun with the baby, have time for yourself, keep the house clean, be involved in the community, work at home or at a job, take care of the rest of your family, and exercise too. But maybe you can't. Please don't despair. Your baby will grow up sooner than you can imagine, and there will be a time when you will once again be able to plan exercise whenever you wish.

What to Do with the Baby While You Exercise
- Hire a baby-sitter.
- Arrange to swap exercise time with another mom. She watches your baby while you exercise and you do the same for her.
- Join a gym that offers childcare services on the premises.
- Exercise while the baby sleeps.
- Put the baby in a swinging seat and let him watch you while you exercise to a tape or TV.
- Get up early and exercise before the baby wakes up.
- Form a new moms' exercise group at home and have one mom care for the babies while the rest of you work out.

EXERCISE GUIDELINES FOR NEW MOTHERS

Since exercise really is different for new mothers, be careful how you start. The following recommendations are based on guidelines put out by the American College of Obstetricians and Gynecologists.

1. Try to exercise three times a week. Competitive sports are discouraged. Swimming, walking, biking, aerobic dancing, and jogging are all acceptable if performed correctly.
2. Do not exercise vigorously in hot, humid weather or if you have a fever.
3. Avoid jerky, bouncy movements; jumping; jarring motions; or activities that require quick changes in direction. Exercise on a wooden floor or a lightly carpeted floor to reduce chances of injury.

4. Warm up before vigorous activity by walking or bicycling on a stationary bike for five minutes.
5. Follow vigorous exercise with a period of gradually declining activity. Because your joints are still somewhat loose after you deliver, don't take stretches to their point of maximum resistance.
6. Check your heart rate by taking your pulse and comparing it to the heart rate guidelines for postpartum mothers listed in the box below. Mothers should not exceed these rates unless they have consulted their doctors.
7. When doing floor exercises, rise from the floor slowly to prevent low blood pressure. Gently exercise your legs following floor exercises.
8. Drink enough fluids to prevent thirst and dehydration.
9. If you were sedentary before you had your baby, begin exercise gradually and advance slowly.

Check Your Pulse

When exercising, checking your pulse will let you know if you are working hard enough to receive health benefits—or if you are working too hard. The chart below lists the target heart rate for postpartum women while exercising. The column on the right lists the number of beats for a ten-second interval. Take your pulse while exercising. If the number of beats exceeds the recommended amount, you are doing too much and should slow down gradually. If your pulse isn't up to the recommended number, pick up the pace a bit and test your pulse again.

Target Heart Rate Guidelines for Postpartum Exercise

Age	Maximum Beats per Minute	Maximum Beats per 10 Seconds *
20	150	25
25	146	24
30	142	23–24
35	138	23

Age	Maximum Beats per Minute	Maximum Beats per 10 Seconds *
40	135	22–23
45	131	22

*Each figure represents 75 percent of the maximum heart rate that would be predicted for the corresponding age group. Under proper medical supervision, more strenuous activity and higher heart rates may be appropriate.

Source: American College of Obstetricians and Gynecologists, *Exercise During Pregnancy and the Postnatal Period*, Home Exercise Program, May 1985, published by the American College of Obstetricians and Gynecologists, Washington, D.C.

ACTIVITIES TO PROMOTE AEROBIC ENDURANCE

Swimming, bicycling, brisk walking, jogging, and aerobic dancing are all good activities for new mothers if the heart-rate guidelines are followed. To get the health benefits of these activities, exercise for fifteen to twenty minutes three times a week.

Since most of us exercise unsupervised and at home, it's important to recognize our bodies' trouble signals. The first rule is that if it hurts, don't do it. If you still believe in the no pain, no gain theory of exercise, you've been misled. The key to successful exercise is consistency. A workout that causes muscle pain, strain, or fatigue can't hold a sweat band to three days of gentle, satisfying brisk walking.

Warning Signs and Symptoms for New Moms

Stop exercising and call your health-care provider if you experience any of the following:

Pain	Faintness
Bleeding	Irregular heartbeats
Dizziness	Back pain
Shortness of breath	Pubic pain
Palpitations	Difficulty walking

WHEN CAN I BEGIN EXERCISE IF I HAD A CESAREAN BIRTH?

This is definitely a question you must ask your doctor. Healing times and medical complications vary from woman to woman. Don't push it. If you feel good and your doctor says you are in good shape and you have the energy, then as early as four weeks postpartum you may be able to begin an appropriate activity. Walking is a good start.

Remember that in addition to having a baby, you had major surgery. Take care of yourself, but don't think of yourself as an invalid either. Appropriate exercise and movement can promote healing and recovery.

WHAT IS A GOOD EXERCISE REGIME?

A good workout program should include exercise that gets your heart up to its target rate, to provide overall conditioning. It's also a good idea to do some abdomen-strengthening exercises, because good strong stomach muscles support your back and can help prevent back injuries.

EXERCISES FOR YOUR ABDOMEN

Pelvic Tilt
1. Stand with your feet shoulder-width apart. Bend your knees slightly.
2. Contract the muscles of your abdomen, buttocks, and pelvis. Gently thrust forward, rotating your pubic bone upward. Imagine that you are moving your pubic bone up toward your navel. Hold this position for ten seconds, then release. Repeat ten times.

This can also be performed while lying down.

Crunches or—The New Safe Sit-up

The sit-up that we all remember from gym class is no longer recommended as an abdomen toner. The old sit-ups only partially exercised the abdominal muscles while putting lots of strain on the back. Performed correctly, the crunch tightens the tummy without hurting the back.

1. Lie on your back, bend your knees, keep your feet on the floor.
2. Put your hands at your sides (you can gently hold on to your thighs) or cross them over your chest. (In time you can increase the difficulty of the crunch by crossing your arms over your head and allowing each hand to gently touch the opposite shoulder.)
3. Contract your stomach muscles, press your lower back into the floor, and lift your upper body up to a thirty-five or forty-five-degree angle.
4. Keep your lower back pressed to the ground without arching and gently return to the floor. Repeat five times. Gently work up to three sets of five.

Many of us perform crunches the wrong way. While "crunching," keep the following in mind:

- To keep your neck properly extended, your chin should not touch your chest. There should always be enough room between chin and chest to fit a fist or an orange there.
- Don't keep your eyes locked on the ceiling. When you're tightening your abdominal muscles and lifting your head, look at your knees. This will help you stay in the correct position.
- Don't forget to breathe and exhale as you lift.
- If you are placing your hands on your chest and your neck feels

tight or strained, place one or both hands under your neck for support.

• Perform crunches in a slow, controlled manner. Fast and jerky is not your goal. This is more like an isometric exercise than an aerobic one.

If the crunch feels too difficult, try the reverse crunch:

1. Sit with your knees bent and reach your arms forward, straight over your knees.
2. Gently lower yourself to the floor. Try to imagine each vertebra making contact with the floor.
3. When you're all the way down, return to the starting position by pushing yourself up with your hands. Repeat this ten times. As you increase abdominal strength, you can start on the regular crunch.

BACK STRENGTHENING

Many mothers have trouble with their backs while pregnant. Exercise now may help prevent future back troubles. The pelvic tilt described in the abdominal exercises is a good back strengthener. There are also some exercises geared specifically to the back.

Lower-Back Stretch

1. Lie on your back.
2. Take hold of one knee with both hands and pull it toward your chin. Keep the other leg on the floor, straight. Count to ten, then switch legs.

The Side-to-Side

1. Lie on your back with your knees slightly bent.
2. Gently drop your knees to the right while turning your body and both arms to the left.

3. Bring your knees to the upright position and drop to the opposite side.

Cat Stretch

1. Get down on all fours, hands and knees shoulder-width apart.
2. Slowly press your navel toward the floor, allowing your lower back to curve down while you lift your head. Return to neutral.
3. Gently arch your back while you lower your head. Return to neutral.
4. Repeat ten times.

STRETCHING GUIDELINES

Maintaining flexibility is a great way to prevent injury. There are many stretches you can perform while doing household activities or watching TV. One of the best books on this subject is *Stretching* by Bob Anderson (Shelter Publications, Inc., 1980).

Here are some guidelines for safe stretching:

- Stop if there's pain.
- Try to stretch three or four times a week.
- Don't bounce when you stretch.
- Hold a stretch in a comfortable position.
- Breathe slowly, and exhale as you begin the stretch.

A NEW MOTHER'S EXERCISE ROUTINE

Here's a sample of a safe, healthy exercise plan for a new mother:

- Monday—Thirty-minute walk (five-minute warm-up, twenty minutes in target heart-rate zone, five-minute cool-down). Stretch.

- Tuesday—Abdomen and back exercises: crunches, pelvic tilt, cat stretch.
- Wednesday—Thirty-minute ride on exercise bike (five-minute warm-up, twenty minutes in target heart rate zone, five-minute cool-down).
- Thursday—Take the day off.
- Friday—Thirty-minute exercise to a video*, TV show, or the ACOG exercise tape. Most exercise programs have the warm-up and cool-down in the workout.
- Saturday and Sunday—Back and abdomen exercises.

Throughout the day, try pulling in your abdomen muscles and holding them for ten seconds. Do this as often as you remember —perhaps each time you change the baby's diaper.

The American College of Obstetricians and Gynecologists has approved and endorsed the *Postnatal Exercise Program* video. See Appendix for details.

IS IT SAFE FOR BREASTFEEDING MOTHERS TO EXERCISE?

This is a good question, since a mother who is quite active can use up calories and may also worry about fatigue. The good news is that exercise appears to be compatible with breastfeeding and may even have some desirable effects on lactation.

Cheryl A. Lovelady, Ph.D., R.D., a nutrition researcher at the University of California, recently studied the impact exercise has on breastfeeding. She and her colleagues recruited sixteen breastfeeding mothers; half were very active, the others were sedentary. Their babies were all between nine and twenty-four weeks old. Each mother was asked to keep a food and activity

---

*Most videotapes and TV exercise shows aren't geared for new mothers, so proceed slowly. When bouncing, jumping exercises are part of the routine, walk in place. New mothers may still have more elasticity in their joints, and too much bouncing could cause injury, so take it easy.

diary. Mothers also collected milk samples for nutrition testing and measured milk volume by using a sophisticated scale to weigh their babies before and after feedings.

The active mothers participated in aerobic activity (usually swimming, but some jogged or biked) five days a week for forty-five minutes. They expended about 3,200 calories daily and ate 2,700. The sedentary mothers ate about 2,100 calories and expended about 2,400 calories while carrying out their usual activities.

The very active mothers experienced no adverse effect on their breastfeeding; in fact, they had higher milk volumes than the sedentary moms. These results suggest that it is fine for new breastfeeding mothers to resume vigorous exercise.

If you exercise regularly and vigorously, you must eat enough to meet the demands of exercise and to produce an adequate supply of breast milk. In most cases, if a mother responds to her appetite and hunger pangs, she'll meet her caloric needs.

Keep in mind that the first four to six weeks are when mother and baby bond and become a nursing couple. Both of you need this time to learn to nurse. For some mothers, a time-consuming vigorous exercise program could compromise this relationship. Use common sense when deciding when to begin your postnatal exercise routine.

PICK A GOOD SPORTS BRA

When engaging in any kind of vigorous activity, wear a sports bra. Choose one made of cotton; synthetic materials can trap moisture and cause irritation. Buy a bra with wide straps and lots of support.

When I was exercising and nursing I found that a sports bra alone didn't do the trick, so I wore two bras. I wore my nursing bra underneath and put the exercise bra on top. This gave me the extra support I needed.

WHAT ABOUT INCLUDING MY BABY IN MY EXERCISE ROUTINE?

In an effort to get exercise, a lot of us are bringing our babies along. Exercise can be a wonderful chance to interact with a baby and expose him to some fresh air and new scenery. Exercising with a baby is not without its downside, however. A June 1990 article in *The Physician and Sportsmedicine* cited the following potential risks associated with including your baby in an exercise routine:

- Swimming classes, even conducted under the watchful eye of a parent and instructor, can allow the baby to consume an excessive and potentially dangerous amount of water. Infants may also pick up intestinal parasites such as giardia or viruses that can be transmitted through pool water. Adults are less susceptible to these invaders than babies.
- Jogging with a baby in a stroller can result in a fall or a collision with other runners, animals, bicycles, or even cars.
- Backpack-type carriers used for jogging may jar and shake a young infant's head, causing brain damage. Even a bike ride over very bumpy terrain is risky with a young infant.
- In chilly weather, a baby joining you in outdoor exercise may become too cold and not be able to communicate the problem to you.
- Exercising in the heat or overexposure to the sun has risks as well, such as sunburn and dehydration.
- Hiking in the wilderness could become a nightmare if emergency help is needed for a serious bug bite or injury.

This all sounds very scary, but you need to be aware of any potential risks if you want to include your baby in your activities. You *can* exercise with your baby, but use good judgment.

In response to the article in *The Physician and Sportsmedicine*, Linda Pescatello, an exercising mom in New Britain, Connecti-

cut, wrote a letter to the editor suggesting the following guidelines for parents who use baby joggers. They sound worthwhile,
so I pass them along to you.

1. Avoid using the jogger during environmental extremes, such
   as hot and humid or cold and blustery weather.
2. Avoid traffic by using the jogger in a park, during a race, or
   in the early morning hours.
3. Avoid bumpy terrain until the baby is at least one year old.
   If rough surfaces are unavoidable, deflate the jogger's tires
   slightly.
4. Use the jogger only when your baby is at least six months
   old.
5. Use a bicycle helmet to protect your baby's head.
6. Use a canopy and sunblock to protect your baby from the
   sun.
7. Never push yourself to exhaustion.

RELAXATION

There's more to good health than just exercising and eating well.
Allowing time for relaxation can go a long way toward promoting well-being. For me, a new baby added quite a bit of stress to
my life. I felt as though I was always rushing to do something
while I managed our home and cared for our family. Relaxation
techniques helped me cope with this stress.

Relaxation therapy isn't really exercise, but it's important to
new mothers. As a breastfeeding mom, you can try some relaxation techniques while you feed the baby. You may both fall
asleep, but that's okay. (If you do tend to fall asleep, you may
want to doze off after you've switched breasts. Otherwise you
may be lopsided from feeding your baby on just one side.) Two
relaxation techniques—imagery and deep breathing—can give
new moms much-needed relief from stress.

Imagery

While you're nursing, make yourself comfortable. Close your eyes and imagine a beautiful scene. Look at every detail. If you're in a garden, look at every flower. Visualize the colors. Imagine how it would feel to walk on soft, cool grass. Imagine how the air would smell. Can you hear birds? Is the sky blue? Are clouds gliding by? Are you sitting or lying down?

Deep Breathing

Make yourself comfortable sitting or lying down, in a position you won't have to move out of too soon. Then take a deep breath, slowly exhale, and breathe in again gently. With each breath you exhale, think of a number (you can count backward or repeat the same number over and over). Continue breathing. Each time you exhale, think of a number and allow the number to push away all other thoughts that try to creep in. Do this for as long as you can. It may be only five minutes. The next day, try it again and see if you can go just a bit longer. If not, that's okay, too. Just that little bit of time you allow your mind to relax can affect your whole body and your well-being.

I FEEL LIKE A FAILURE

For lots of us, exercise is an all-or-nothing commitment. We set goals for exercising three to four times a week, we meet these goals for a week or two, and then we stop. Our usual response is that we failed. We feel guilty, and that's the end of the exercise program—until we get concerned again about our weight or health and make new commitments, carry them out for a week or two, and let them too fall by the wayside.

Here's my advice: assume that your exercise routine will always be in transition and that there will be weeks when you meet all your goals and weeks when you won't. Just keep doing it. You aren't a failure because you didn't exercise.

SPEAK POSITIVELY

You aren't alone if the desire to exercise doesn't come naturally. Over my career as a dietitian I have talked to literally thousands of people about exercising more. It is a rare client who approaches exercise with enthusiasm. Most of the time I hear comments like "I know I should, but I just can't find the time." Instead of thinking of exercise as an additional burden, try to see it as a privilege. Start speaking positively about it and tell friends and family: "Boy, I love to get out and take my walks" or "It feels so good to get out and move" or "Gee, since I started to exercise more I really do feel better."

Try speaking and thinking positively about exercising, and you may even find it's more of a pleasure than a burden.

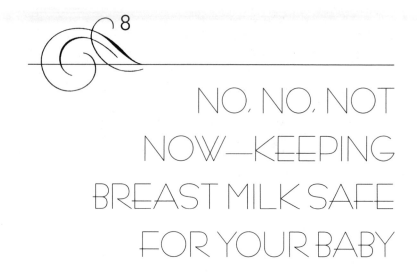

NO, NO, NOT NOW—KEEPING BREAST MILK SAFE FOR YOUR BABY

AS NEW PARENTS WE PAY ATTENTION TO EVERY LITTLE BURP, coo, and cry our babies make. It's likely that while you're breast-feeding, you'll be more concerned with what you eat than at any other time in your life. Breastfeeding moms almost always try to analyze how meals affect their babies. If the baby is up at night the mom blames the spicy spaghetti sauce at dinner or the chocolate bar she snacked on after lunch.

When our babies are fussy or crying we try to determine what we ate that we shouldn't have so that we can remove the offending substance from our diets. The truth is that little babies cry and they cry and then they cry some more. Most of the time our babies cry in reaction to something completely unrelated to what we have eaten. But sometimes, what we eat does affect how our babies feel.

Concern about eating well while breastfeeding is indeed a

good thing, but don't be too hard on yourself. Some mothers won't go near a cup of coffee, or they completely restrict the salt and spices in their food. This chapter will explore the facts behind the food myths that have surrounded the diets of breast-feeding mothers for generations. In most cases, moderation is the key to a happy mother and a happy baby. But there are some things moms do need to be cautious about, including caffeine, alcohol, drugs, and pesticides.

CAN I EAT IT?

It's not uncommon to gather with a group of nursing mothers for lunch and hear questions about the menu like "What's in it?" "Does it have garlic?" "Are there onions in this?"

It's true that what we eat affects our health and breast milk, but there is no scientific evidence that foods that cause gas in you create gas in your baby. Even if you eat a big bowl of beans and feel discomfort yourself, the gas in your intestinal tract does not go into your bloodstream and it does not get into your breast milk. Foods that give you gas aren't going to do the same for your baby.

Foods like oranges, grapefruit, or tomatoes are often thought of as too acid for a baby. Again, there's no evidence to support this. Once you eat an acidic food, it mixes with your digestive juices and reaches the pH (acid level) that's right for your body. An acidic food cannot change the pH of your blood or your breast milk.

A complex system of checks and balances keeps your body in harmony even when you eat large servings of certain foods. Yes, you may find that some foods eaten by you do affect the baby. If so, eliminate the food and try it again a week or so later. If it bothers the baby again, stay away from it. If it doesn't bother the baby again, the connection the first time around may have just been a coincidence.

There is no harm in eliminating or temporarily avoiding a few foods while you breastfeed. The danger comes only if you eliminate whole food groups such as dairy, citrus fruits, or wheat products.

One recent and fascinating report might actually encourage mothers to try more flavorful foods. Researcher Dr. Julie Mennella at the Monell Chemical Senses Center in Philadelphia asked eight breastfeeding mothers to eat garlic extract capsules before nursing their babies. The capsules significantly changed the odor of the mothers' milk. Instead of the garlic being a deterrent, the babies actually nursed longer and consumed more milk than they did when their mothers ate a relatively bland diet. This research suggests that flavorful foods should not be eliminated from the breastfeeding mother's menu. In fact, the researchers speculate that early exposure to a variety of flavors in breast milk may increase a baby's willingness to try a greater variety of foods as a child.

Almost all the reports of foods eaten by a mother affecting her baby are anecdotal stories; I couldn't find any hard research evidence. In Dr. Ruth Lawrence's excellent book *Breastfeeding: A Guide for the Medical Profession,* she reports that the natural oils in some foods such as garlic and some spices have flavors and odors that might be capable of passing into breast milk and upsetting a baby. Garlic, onions, cabbage, turnips, broccoli, dried beans, rhubarb, apricots, and prunes are all mentioned by Dr. Lawrence as potential causes of colic, as is a heavy diet of fresh fruits and melons. There are no studies that I know of to support this assertion, but these foods are commonly cited by mothers as being troublesome. Since I trust the collective wisdom of experienced moms, I suspect there is probably some validity to the list. Mothers know their bodies best. Just don't be a slave to what works for other women.

Dr. Lawrence described another interesting effect food can have on breast milk. One mother's breast milk turned pink-orange from the dyes used in the orange soda she routinely drank. Other mothers have reported green milk from drinking Gatorade, taking some medications, or eating kelp, other seaweeds, and certain vitamins from the health-food store. To get rid of an unusual color, the mother's diet must be scrutinized and the coloring agent avoided. No health risks to the baby from colored milk are known, but certainly it's best to avoid these chemicals.

CAN I DRINK COFFEE?

When I first started to nurse Sarah, one of the first changes I made in my diet was to eliminate regular coffee. The caffeine in coffee is a stimulant, and I didn't want Sarah to be any more wakeful, particularly at night, than she already was. Much later, when I started to research some of the particulars about what mothers should and should not eat, I found that caffeine, in small amounts, wasn't that bad. But it can pose a problem if consumed in large amounts.

One cup of regular coffee won't harm your baby. Your body quickly absorbs the 150 milligrams of caffeine in a cup of coffee, but only about 1 to 5 milligrams of that caffeine will end up in a full liter of your breast milk. This is a very small amount, but there is a catch. In the adult body, caffeine stays in the bloodstream for only three to five hours before it's excreted. It can remain in your baby's blood for eighty hours—up to ninety-seven hours for preterm infants. This means that infants can accumulate caffeine. One cup of coffee a day shouldn't cause trouble, but a mother drinking more than three cups a day may start to have an irritable, wakeful baby.

Caffeine is not only found in coffee (table 8). Tea and dark colas can be significant caffeine sources if you drink them frequently.

Table 8. Caffeine Content of Selected Beverages and Foods

Coffee—5 ounces	
Brewed drip	130 mg
Percolator	94 mg
Instant	74 mg
Decaffeinated	3 mg
Tea—5 ounces	
Brewed, U.S. brands	40 mg
Brewed, imported	60 mg
Iced tea—12 ounces	70 mg
Colas—12 ounces	
Regular	30–46 mg
Diet	2–58 mg
Caffeine free	0–trace
Jolt	72 mg
Fresca, 7-Up, Sprite, Squirt—12 ounces	0 mg
Cocoa—5 ounces	4 mg
Chocolate milk—8 oz	5 mg
Dark chocolate—1 ounce	20 mg
Milk chocolate—1 ounce	6 mg

Switching to decaffeinated coffee can certainly reduce your caffeine intake, but it doesn't seem to be just the caffeine in coffee that's the problem. A 1989 study of breastfeeding mothers drinking more than three cups of coffee per day while they were pregnant and breastfeeding found that the concentrations of iron in the mothers' breast milk was low and their babies' own iron status was compromised. Coffee's effect on iron doesn't seem to be linked to caffeine but to some other chemical component.

Because of coffee's adverse effects on breastfeeding babies, it's best if you drink only one to two cups a day and keep your total daily caffeine intake below 300 milligrams.

CHOCOLATE—THE FOOD WE HATE OURSELVES FOR LOVING

Chocolate is surrounded by folklore. Mothers who eat chocolate while breastfeeding fear they'll give their babies diarrhea, irritability, even eczema. Though there are many anecdotal reports about how chocolate is thought to affect babies, hard evidence is scarce.

One 1977 study seems to take chocolate off the breastfeeding mothers' no list. Beth Resman, Pharm.D., a researcher at the State University of New York at Buffalo, asked six breastfeeding mothers to eat a single 4-ounce serving of Hershey's milk chocolate. She found that none of the infants in her study experienced any adverse effect when their mothers ate this moderate portion of chocolate. If you love chocolate, go ahead and eat small amounts—I don't want you to feel deprived, and your baby probably won't mind. But if you are convinced that chocolate bothers your baby, then by all means stay away from it. Chocolate has no redeeming nutritional value. It just tastes good.

Why Do We Love Chocolate?

Many women complain of being chocoholics, particularly around their periods. There may be some scientific reason for this. It seems that our need for calories increases during our menstrual cycle, and binging on chocolate, a concentrated source of calories, may be a way to meet that need.

Chocolate may also act like a mood-altering drug. It's rich in substances that raise our spirits and make us feel better. I know chocolate makes me feel better. I love the way it tastes and smells. I also know that it's rich in fat and calories, so I don't even keep it in the house. My compromise is to treat myself on special occasions to some sort of chocolate that I really enjoy: homemade chocolate sauce is my usual choice. You can try the fat-free chocolate sauce I use as my occasional treat—the recipe is on page 187.

If heartburn is a problem for you, chocolate might be a food to avoid. Chocolate and other foods such as alcohol, coffee, spearmint, peppermint, and those with high fat are thought to increase heartburn symptoms.

IS IT SAFE TO TAKE MEDICATION WHILE BREASTFEEDING?

Don't take any medications unless you absolutely must. Many drugs pass into breast milk; some could cause your child discomfort or even harm. Always check with your physician before taking any prescription or over-the-counter medication.

If you must take a prescription medication, have a frank discussion with your doctor. Make sure he knows you're breastfeeding. If he doesn't know what effect the drug might have on your nursing baby, then ask him to gather additional information from one of the medical hotlines he is sure to be familiar with.

If you must take medication, it may be best to take it right after your baby has nursed. This way the medication may no longer be as active in your bloodstream and breast milk by the next feeding.

IS IT SAFE TO DRINK ALCOHOL WHILE BREASTFEEDING?

Your own common sense will have already told you that heavy drinking is absolutely unacceptable while breastfeeding.

The alcohol you drink passes from your stomach to your bloodstream. If you drink only a small amount, your liver can quickly remove the alcohol from your blood. But if you drink a lot, your liver can't keep up, and your blood levels will get even higher with each sip. The alcohol in your blood can pass into your breast milk. If there's a lot of alcohol in your blood, then not only do you get drunk—so does your baby.

Besides causing drunkenness, excess alcohol can interfere with oxytocin, the chemical that controls milk ejection. Excess alcohol consumption can thus slow the delivery of milk to your baby.

Okay, so you know that getting drunk isn't advised, but what about a glass of wine with supper? It has long been thought that the occasional glass of wine or cold beer can help a mother relax and thus actually assist in the letdown reflex and breastfeeding itself. Studies have shown that within thirty minutes of drinking a small amount of alcohol, especially beer, a mother's levels of prolactin, the hormone that stimulates milk production, increase significantly.

The Subcommittee on Nutrition During Lactation suggests that mothers who want to drink while breastfeeding consume not more than 2 to 2.5 ounces of liquor, 8 ounces of wine, or two cans of beer in any one day. These guidelines are designed to protect your baby from becoming intoxicated, but you must remember that a couple of beers each night is going to add a few hundred extra calories (table 9) and the alcohol is likely to leave you quite groggy at that two o'clock feeding.

Table 9. Calorie Content of Various Alcoholic Beverages

Regular beer—12 ounces	151 calories
Light beer—12 ounces	100 calories*
80-proof liquor—1.5 ounces	97 calories
White wine—7 ounces	174 calories

*This is an estimate. Individual products may vary in caloric content.

When I first began to investigate what mothers should eat and drink while breastfeeding, I was told by one prominent doctor that there was absolutely no evidence that one alcoholic drink consumed by a nursing mother would harm a healthy baby. That was in 1987. Since then, a cloud of suspicion has been cast over the safety of that one drink.

Dr. Ruth Little of the University of Michigan studied four

hundred infants to investigate the effects a mother's moderate alcohol intake had on her year-old infant. Dr. Little found that tests designed to measure mental function did not uncover any connection between what the mother drank and how her breastfed baby fared on the test. However, the children whose mothers had at least one drink daily, did score lower on motor-development tests than infants who were not exposed to as much alcohol.

The study didn't consider the actual amount of alcohol in the breast milk, socioeconomic variables, or the way the mothers interacted with their children, but it does seem to link moderate maternal alcohol consumption with impaired motor development in children.

Mothers, Lead, and Wine

Foil-wrapped wines may be a source of lead for mothers-to-be and nursing mothers. According to the Food and Drug Administration, foil wrappers can leave lead-salt deposits on a bottle's rim. These deposits are dissolved when the wine is poured. Once a woman drinks the wine, she could pass the lead to her growing fetus or nursing infant. To reduce this risk, wipe the rim of the bottle, as well as the exposed cork, with a cloth moistened with lemon, vinegar, or water before pouring. Of course the surefire way to avoid the lead is to avoid the wines with this type of wrapper.

In a more recent 1991 study in the *New England Journal of Medicine*, Julie Mennella, Ph.D., and Gary Beauchamp, Ph.D., asked twelve nursing mothers to drink orange juice mixed with a small amount of alcohol. The researchers compared how the babies nursed after the alcoholic drink to how they nursed after their mothers drank a glass of plain orange juice. The babies consumed significantly less milk after their mothers drank the orange juice with alcohol. The researchers suspect that alcohol may have an undesirable effect on the flavor of breast milk, diminish a baby's ability or desire to feed, or even decrease milk production.

Sensory tests conducted on the mothers' milk showed that a change in odor peaked thirty to sixty minutes after they drank the alcohol. This suggests that mothers who know they will be drinking may want to feed their babies before having that drink. Alcohol, whether it is wine, beer, or liquor, must be consumed cautiously by breastfeeding mothers. It provides calories and if consumed in excess could harm you and upset your baby. So if you choose to drink, do so in moderation.

ILLEGAL DRUGS

The prudent thing to do while breastfeeding is to avoid all drugs, including marijuana and cocaine. The active ingredient in marijuana is tetrahydrocannabinol; once absorbed, this chemical is stored in body fat. Since body fat is used to fuel breast-milk production, a mother who is a heavy marijuana user may have marijuana in her milk. A child ingesting marijuana from breast milk may appear more sleepy and become less interested in nursing. Animal studies show that newborn animals drinking mother's milk contaminated with marijuana had alterations in their brain cells. Since your marijuana smoking can have a negative impact on your baby, please don't smoke during the months you breastfeed. Not only can the chemicals harm your baby directly —if you smoke, you won't be fully alert to your baby's needs, either.

If a mother uses cocaine or heroin it can show up in her milk. Though there are no studies on the effect these drugs have on nursing infants, it is known that during pregnancy both drugs can have serious negative consequences for the developing baby such as low birth weight. Common sense should be your guide. Mothers who can't stop using these substances should stop nursing.

Marijuana, alcohol, heroin, and cocaine do more than affect

your body. They affect your mind and your judgment. A baby needs your unclouded attention, and a new mother just can't be at her best if any of these drugs are in the way.

WILL CIGARETTE SMOKE HURT MY BABY?

Cigarette smoking is actively discouraged because of its effect on you and your baby. If you quit smoking while pregnant, please don't take it up again. Once your baby is delivered it might not seem so important not to smoke, but it still is.

First of all, smoking hurts you. Heavy smokers have more lung and heart disease. The nicotine from cigarettes may also pass into your breast milk and upset your baby. A mother who smokes twenty cigarettes a day can have a high level of fat-soluble nicotine in her breast milk, which could cause nausea and vomiting in her baby. Cigarette smoking can also reduce milk volume, because it inhibits prolactin and oxytocin production. Babies with mothers who smoke tend to be weaned sooner and have a greater incidence of colic.

Finally, there is the real problem of secondhand smoke. Even formula-fed babies exposed to secondhand smoke have measurable levels of nicotine in their urine, meaning they are inhaling the cigarette smoke along with the smoker. A child who breathes in a smoke-filled environment may have more respiratory problems.

Infrequent smoking is probably okay, but mothers who smoke ten to twenty cigarettes or more each day should definitely quit or try to cut down. At the very least don't smoke around your baby. Don't let visitors smoke around your baby either.

A child in a smoking household is more likely to come across matches or lighters that look like toys and are capable of causing serious burns. Parents who smoke can accidently burn their child with falling ashes. A child may see a lit cigarette and reach for it out of curiosity with disastrous results. And if mom and dad smoke, then their child may start the same unhealthy habit when he reaches adolescence.

THE HIDDEN MENACE

As a mother, the dangers that worry me the most are the ones I can't see. Pesticides alarm us because most of us don't understand how they work. And, worst of all, we can't control them. Scientists try to reassure us that the foods we eat are safe, even if they contain pesticides. As a breastfeeding mother, you may feel that your baby is safe from environmental contaminants because he has not yet started on food. The sad truth is that almost all mothers carry contaminants such as PCBs and dioxin in their bodies. Our babies may even have been exposed to the chemicals as we carried them in our wombs. This exposure probably continues as we breastfeed.

Dioxin is a byproduct of chemical manufacturing and incineration. You may be most familiar with this chemical as the contaminant in Agent Orange, the defoliant used in Vietnam. Dioxin has been accumulating in dirt, riverbeds, and on plants since the 1940s. It accumulates particularly well in fat. When we eat the fish that feed in the rivers or the animals that eat the dioxin-tainted plant foods or the grains grown in soil with dioxin in it, then we ingest the dioxin, too. That dioxin can pass into our breast milk.

The debate continues as to the risk to babies drinking breast milk contaminated with dioxin. One article cited the risks from drinking dioxin-tainted breast milk as minuscule when compared to the risk associated with riding in a car. Commercial formula is virtually dioxin free, but it doesn't offer the health-promoting benefits of breastfeeding and is not recommended as an alternative.

Since dioxin accumulates in fat and other tissues, the best a mother can do is to control her own animal-fat intake and lose weight slowly. Since milk is in part synthesized from the mother's own stored fat supplies, it is thought that rapid weight loss may increase the concentration of the chemical in her milk. The truth is that we don't know if weight loss results in more chemicals in breast milk or if it allows the body to excrete these chemicals through feces or urine. Prudent weight loss of no more than four and a half pounds a month is probably the best path.

In a study published in the *American Journal of Public Health,* Dr. Walter Rogan found that the presence of some chemicals in breast milk may interfere with the length of time a mother breastfeeds. Dr. Rogan began a project in 1978 that measured the content of polychlorinated biphenyls (PCBs) and dichlorodiphenyl dichloroethene (DDE, a metabolite of the infamous DDT pesticide) being consumed by 858 children who were breastfed by their mothers. Dr. Rogan found that women with higher concentrations of DDE and perhaps PCBs breastfed for a shorter length of time. DDE may have an estrogen-like effect that suppresses lactation.

This study was not designed to investigate the children's long-term cancer risk, but they remain under surveillance and more information may be available with time. The good news is that the children exposed to high levels of DDE or PCBs didn't show any adverse effects on growth, health, or weight gain or impact on how often they went to see the doctor for illness.

To reduce your risk of undesirable chemical and pesticide ingestion and minimize your baby's exposure to these substances, you can

- Eat a wide variety of foods so that you limit your exposure from any one food.
- Try to buy foods in season, which can mean they have fewer chemicals on them.
- But low-fat dairy products.
- Trim all meats.
- Don't eat poultry skin.
- Bake or broil instead of frying.

- Eat lots of fruits and vegetables.
- Buy local produce or at least produce grown in the United States.
- Wash your produce; submerge in water and scrub with a vegetable brush.
- Peel waxed foods like cucumbers, peppers, and apples.
- If using orange or lemon peel or zest in a recipe, buy organic fruit.
- Discard outer leaves of cabbage.
- If your diet is already rich in fiber, peel carrots, peaches, and pears.
- If you buy organic, ask the produce manager what the term means. There is not yet a legal definition of "organic," though it is usually thought to mean that the foods were grown without the use of pesticides.

Ask your supermarket to label the origins of the foods it sells. If they're not labeled, ask the produce manager where the food comes from. He'll know if the fruits and vegetables are from Naples, Florida, or Naples, Italy. Foods grown within the United States must comply with U.S. guidelines for pesticide use, and these products are often better regulated than produce from foreign countries.

For more information on pesticides and food safety look in the Resources section at the end of the book.

Let common sense guide you when making decisions about what you will put in your mouth. Alcohol, drugs, and too much caffeine could all be passed on to your baby. While breastfeeding, you must be cautious. There are still plenty of good foods and nonalcoholic drinks to be enjoyed so you won't feel deprived.

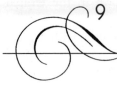

SPECIAL PROBLEMS— SPECIFIC ANSWERS

CESAREAN BIRTH, RETURNING TO WORK, DIABETES, VEGETARIAN menus, allergies, anemias, hemorrhoids, and premature births are just a few of the issues that breastfeeding mothers may have to deal with. Eating properly can help a mother cope successfully with these special situations.

ALLERGIES

Fifteen percent of North Americans have some form of allergic disease ranging from mild skin rash to life-threatening asthma. If you have a family history of allergies, your decision to breast-feed is a good one. Breastfeeding alone doesn't guarantee that your child won't get an allergy, but it does appear to reduce the risk and postpone onset. Breast milk may protect babies against allergies by boosting their immune systems, and mothers may be able to pass on some of their own allergy-fighting substances to their babies in their milk. A baby is most likely to develop a food allergy when she is between four and nine months old. By breastfeeding and delaying the introduction of solid foods until a child is four to six months old, you will reduce her chance of developing a food allergy. Protein is the substance in food that triggers an allergic reaction. For this reason, supplemental protein foods are not needed or recommended until a baby is eight or nine months old. Breast milk supplies plenty of protein for young infants and babies.

Foods Most Likely to Cause Allergies	
Eggs	Wheat
Milk and other dairy products	Fish
Peanuts	Chicken
Soybeans	

Since the late 1970s, researchers have been investigating whether the foods a mother eats can help prevent allergies in her child. Several studies are now available that demonstrate that what a breastfeeding mother eats can affect her child's risk for allergies. Proteins are common allergy offenders. The protein a mother eats may cross over into the milk she produces and precipitate an allergic reaction in her baby.

In a study by Ranjit Chandra, M.D., published in *Clinical Allergy*, 109 mothers completed a research project that followed them through pregnancy and lactation. All the mothers had an older child with an allergy or eczema. Half were assigned a diet that restricted their intake of potentially problematic foods such as dairy products, eggs, fish, beef, and peanuts. The other half were given no food restrictions.

Dr. Chandra confirmed that mothers avoiding the common allergenic foods during pregnancy and lactation had children with a lower incidence of allergies and less severe cases of allergic disease. Children of the women on the restricted diet had fewer incidences of eczema; when it did occur, the eczema was milder than that of the children whose mothers did not restrict their diets. Even the babies born to mothers who followed the restricted diet while pregnant but chose formula over breast milk had less severe cases of eczema.

Before you mothers with family histories of allergies start restricting every potentially problematic food, we have to look beyond the study group and statistics to see how this translates to individuals. Of the fifty-five mothers on the avoidance diet, seventeen had babies who developed eczema; of the fifty-four mothers on the regular diet, twenty-four had babies who developed eczema. Statistically, there is a measurable difference in these two groups, but the restricted diet didn't eliminate the risk of allergy. Even though this study and others like it show that a percentage of mothers and babies may be helped by a restricted diet, that diet will not benefit all mothers and their babies.

Imagine too how difficult it would be to avoid eggs, dairy products, and beef. Also think of the changes in the nutritional quality of your diet if you eliminated these protein-rich foods. Of course if it would protect your baby against a lifelong battle with allergies, I know you're thinking it might be worth it.

The Subcommittee on Nutrition During Lactation advises mothers not to eliminate whole food groups to treat allergy unless there is evidence that the mother is "sensitive or intolerant to the food or that the breastfed infant reacts to the food ingested by the mother."

A mother who suspects her breastfed baby is allergic to a particular food she's eating may want to try an elimination diet under the supervision of her doctor. In this case the offending food is taken out of the mother's diet to see if the baby's symptoms disappear. Then the food is reintroduced under careful supervision to determine whether the symptoms reappear. If they do, the culprit has been exposed. If the food must be eliminated for weeks or months, then the mother will have to do some special dietary planning. For example, if she must eliminate eggs she can make up for the lost protein by substituting meat, cheese, or fish. A diet void of all the potentially problematic foods is not recommended on a preventative basis for mothers because it is not found to help all babies, and it could compromise their nutritional status.

CAN I CONTROL COLIC BY WHAT I EAT?

Colic is one of the most frustrating problems parents have with infants. It affects about 20 percent of all babies. For no reason that can be determined, a happy, smiling baby starts to cry. His legs pull up, fists clench, his face turns red, and he screams in pain for an hour or more. As quickly as it starts, it can stop. Holding the baby upright or laying him, tummy side down, on a warm water bottle may help. Often, nothing works to calm him except time. These crying bouts seem to occur most frequently in the late afternoon or early evening, usually when a baby is between six weeks and three months old.

No one knows for sure, but these crying jags may be caused by an immaturity in a baby's newly working digestive tract that can cause spasm or cramps. There is a lot of talk about how a mother's diet can affect colic symptoms but not a lot of research. Dr. Irene Jakobsson from the University of Lund in Sweden has published two studies on this problem.

In her first study published in 1978 in *The Lancet*, Dr. Jakobsson asked eighteen mothers with colicky babies to eat a milk-free diet. Almost immediately the colic disappeared in thirteen of the babies; symptoms reappeared in twelve of the babies when their mothers started drinking milk again. In a later study published in the journal *Pediatrics*, Dr. Jakobsson studied sixty-six mothers and their colicky babies. Again she found that when mothers were put on a milk-free diet, the colic disappeared in thirty-five of the breastfed infants, reappearing in twenty-three of those infants when their mothers started drinking milk again.

Dr. Jacobsson has concluded that in one-third of breastfed infants, colic is related to cow's milk consumption by the mother and that when colic is a problem, mothers should try a milk-free diet. It is believed that part of the cow's milk protein that the mother drinks passes into her breast milk. Some infants may have trouble digesting this form of protein, and colic is the result.

A very recent study sheds even more light on cow's milk and colic. Dr. Patrick Clyne and Dr. Anthony Kulczycki reported in the journal *Pediatrics* on their study of twenty-nine mothers of colicky babies and thirty mothers with babies the same age who did not have colic. The mothers who had colicky babies had much higher levels of cow antibodies in their breast milk than the other mothers. These antibodies are proteins that occur in small amounts in cow's milk. Until this study, only the larger proteins in cow's milk had been examined as a cause of colic. It appears that the more milk a mother drinks, the more cow's milk antibodies she will ingest and pass on to her baby through her own milk. Cow's milk antibodies can also be found in formula made from cow's milk. This helps to explain why colic is more likely to occur in a bottle-fed baby than a breastfed baby.

Why all babies don't get colic and why only some are helped when their mother stops drinking cow's milk is unknown. Colic probably has other causes, including psychological ones. So don't just worry about what you're eating; give some good old-fashioned hugs and cuddles, too. It never hurts to reassure and comfort a child. And whatever you do, or don't do, your baby will probably outgrow colic symptoms by the time he's three months old.

SHOULD I STOP DRINKING MILK?

There just isn't enough evidence to make an across-the-board recommendation that mothers should reduce their cow's milk consumption to avoid or eliminate colic. If colic is a problem, a temporary elimination of milk can be tried. If Dr. Jakobsson is right that 30 percent of colicky breastfed babies can get relief if their mothers eliminate milk, then it's worth a try. The colic should correct itself by the time your baby is three months old, at which time you can start eating milk products again.

The problem with eliminating milk is that it puts you at even greater risk of not meeting your calcium needs. After all, it's difficult for mothers to meet the calcium recommendation even if they are milk drinkers. Mothers avoiding dairy products may need to discuss calcium supplements with their doctors.

IF I CAN'T DRINK MILK, WHAT SHOULD I DO?

Some mothers can't drink milk. They may have a milk allergy or an inability to digest the milk sugar called lactose. If lactose intolerance is your problem, you can find help by using Lactaid, an over-the-counter product that contains an enzyme that pre-digests lactose so that you don't have to. Lactaid milk and cheeses, which are as rich in calcium and protein as regular cow's milk products, are also available (look in the Resources section for suggestions on where to find Lactaid products). Lactaid milk and cheeses still contain cow's milk proteins, so they are not products for people with milk allergies.

Mothers who are allergic to milk or who are on a self-imposed milk-free diet must do some careful planning. A milk-free diet means no yogurt, cheese, ice cream, buttermilk, or cottage cheese, which eliminates some of your very best calcium sources. These mothers will need to eat lots of nondairy calcium-rich foods (table 10) or take an appropriate supplement.

Table 10. Calcium-Rich Nondairy Foods

The following foods, in the portions listed, provide 300 milli-grams of calcium, as much as is contained in 1 cup of milk. The RDA for lactating women is 1,200 milligrams of calcium a day.

Food	Portion providing 300 mg calcium
Sardines with bones	3 ounces
Spinach	1¾ cups cooked
Oysters	6–9 medium
Turnip greens	1¼ cups cooked
Broccoli	2¼ cups cooked
Salmon, canned, with bones	1 cup
Beet greens	2 cups cooked
Dandelion greens	2 cups cooked
Soybeans	2 cups cooked
Tofu	8 ounces
Collards	¾ cup cooked
Almonds	1 cup chopped

Milk doesn't just provide calcium. It is also a good source of protein, vitamin D, and some of the B vitamins. Be cautious if you consider eliminating it from your diet.

SHOULD I TAKE CALCIUM SUPPLEMENTS?

Calcium supplements fall woefully short on nutrition when compared to milk. They contain only calcium and none of the other nutrients found in milk. Calcium in pills is also not as well absorbed as dietary calcium. But if calcium pills are needed, there are a few things you should know.

Calcium carbonate is the least expensive form of this nutrient, and it is one of the more concentrated supplement sources. This is important because if supplements are your primary source of calcium, you will need to take enough to meet your goal of 1,200 milligrams every day. Regular multivitamin-mineral preparations don't contain this large amount. Multivitamin-mineral supplements are not a recommended way to get the calcium you need because you would probably need to take quite a few of the pills, and then your intake of other nutrients like zinc and vitamins A, D, and B₆ might be excessive.

Many women have turned to the antacid Tums as an inexpensive and easy way to get calcium. Tums is calcium carbonate, and though it is marketed as a medicine, it is a safe and reliable way to supplement your diet with calcium. One Tums tablet contains 200 to 300 milligrams of calcium.

The dosage you need will depend on how many foods with calcium you eat. If you don't eat dairy but eat lots of calcium-rich green leafy vegetables or tofu, you may not need to take a full 1,200 milligrams of calcium pills a day. In most cases, the only mothers who need to be careful of calcium supplementation are those who are prone to kidney stones. If kidney stones have plagued you, talk over the use of calcium pills with your doctor. Any mother taking calcium supplements should drink plenty of fluids. This keeps your urine diluted and reduces your risk for kidney stones. You may be able to enhance the absorption of the calcium in your pills by spreading them out through the day instead of taking one large dose.

Calcium-fortified orange juice, bread, cereals, and even soft drinks are now available in most supermarkets. These foods can boost calcium intake, but the calcium in these products may not be well absorbed.

The Subcommittee on Nutrition During Lactation recommends that mothers who cannot eat milk, cheese, or other dairy products and cannot eat enough of alternative calcium nondairy foods should take a supplement of 600 milligrams of elemental calcium per day with meals. At this dosage, calcium is safe. Long-term intake of calcium above 2,500 milligrams daily has not been studied and should be avoided.

CESAREAN

In 1989 (the most recent year for which data are available) 23.8 percent of births in the United States were cesareans. At one time, it was thought that once a mother had a cesarean birth all her subsequent deliveries would have to be cesareans. Today, there is a strong movement to encourage mothers to have vaginal births after cesareans. Because of this shift in medical thinking the number of cesarean sections will probably decline.

A cesarean birth can have both pluses and minuses for breastfeeding mothers. The minuses are that it is major surgery, requires medication, can be quite uncomfortable, and calls for additional recuperation time. In most cases, mothers can see their baby immediately after she is born, but they are usually not able to hold or nurse the child right away. A mother in pain may be less able to focus on her new baby. A cesarean birth also means a woman must adjust to her new role as a mother while she recovers from surgery—a double whammy.

So what are the pluses? Of course, the big plus is that cesarean birth can save the life of mother and baby. Mothers usually stay in the hospital longer, and for first-time moms this can be a real help. Mothers who leave after three days, which is usually the case with vaginal births, won't have the support of the medical staff and the intelligent OB nurses to answer their questions when the baby "wakes up" and really starts to nurse. In this mother's opinion, it is when the milk comes in a few days after delivery that new mothers start to worry about such problems as sore nipples and their ability to breastfeed. Mothers with C-sections are still in the hospital when this happens and they can get lots of professional assistance and support to help them be more confident about their decision to breastfeed.

A cesarean birth rarely interferes with the breastfeeding experience. Delaying nursing would only be necessary if the baby is ill or the mother has medical complications. If the baby cannot be nursed soon after a cesarean birth, then arrangements should be made for the mother to use a breast pump every three hours until she and her baby can be united.

Mothers who had cesarean births need the same nutrients as any new mother but probably a few more calories for the first few weeks because of the extra energy required to heal their wounds. Vitamin C and zinc are two nutrients that promote wound healing, so make sure you get a good vitamin C food daily and select some foods such as crabmeat, beef, liver, eggs, chicken, and whole-wheat bread for zinc.

Constipation can be a problem after surgery, and some extra high-fiber cereal, whole grain breads, and whole fruits may be helpful. You should also drink enough fluids, which can help with constipation and help prevent a urinary-tract infection (these are more likely after a cesarean birth because a catheter is placed in the bladder during surgery).

CHOLESTEROL

In the late 1980s, the National Heart, Lung, and Blood Institute started an all-out campaign to bring cholesterol to our attention. As a result, our cholesterol levels are routinely measured during physicals, and much of America is trying to follow a diet that is lower in cholesterol. Many breastfeeding mothers have questions about cholesterol. For instance, can a mother safely adhere to a low-cholesterol diet while breastfeeding? Should a mother restrict cholesterol while breastfeeding? Can her diet affect the cholesterol in her breast milk and hurt or improve her baby's own cholesterol level?

Cholesterol is a fat that we make in our livers and consume in food. It is present in every body tissue. Only animal foods contain cholesterol; fruits, vegetables, and grains are cholesterol free. Cholesterol is now considered unhealthy, but that's not true. We need cholesterol. It makes up part of some essential hormones and tissues. What *is* harmful is an excessive blood level of the stuff. When blood cholesterol levels are too high, the risk for heart disease is thought to increase.

Naturally, researchers and mothers would like to know just how to start infants off on the right dietary path to avoid a cholesterol problem in adulthood. Though the subject has been studied quite a bit, the answers are still inconclusive.

Research suggests that a rise in cholesterol level may be a natural part of pregnancy and lactation. In a 1985 Swedish study reported in *Obstetrics and Gynecology*, mothers had higher cholesterol levels eight weeks after they gave birth than they did before conception.

Breastfeeding mothers tend to have higher cholesterol levels than mothers who aren't nursing. In a study conducted by Dr. R. H. Knopp that compared the cholesterol levels of new mothers, the lactating mothers had a mean cholesterol level of 207, while the women who were not breastfeeding had a mean cholesterol level of 188. This is a significant difference. A desirable cholesterol level is thought to be less than 200 milligrams per deciliter. A reading between 200 and 239 is said to be borderline high.

In this study, the breastfeeding mothers might have had a total cholesterol level that was technically borderline, but their mean level of "good cholesterol," or HDL, was 65; other mothers had a mean of only 51. The more HDL we have in our blood the better, because HDL seems to help carry the "bad cholesterol," or LDL, out of our bodies. In this study, the levels of HDL were in the healthy range for both the nursing and the bottle-feeding mothers, but it's nice to know that the breastfeeding moms had a higher level of HDL, which many nutritionists think protects against atherosclerosis, or clogged arteries.

There is no evidence that mothers can increase or decrease the cholesterol content of their breast milk by altering what they eat. The cholesterol content of your milk will stay remarkably constant in the range of 100 to 150 milligrams per liter of milk no matter what you eat. This is true even if you have a very high level of blood cholesterol yourself. You wouldn't want to decrease the cholesterol in your baby's milk anyway. Cholesterol is essential to the newborn. She needs it for proper brain development and for the protection of nerve cells.

Breast milk has a higher cholesterol content than formula. Researchers have been trying to determine if this is desirable or not. Some evidence obtained from animal studies suggests that breastfed babies may be at an advantage. By consuming more cholesterol as infants, they may be able to handle cholesterol better as adults. This issue is complex; for now, study results remain inconclusive.

While a mother's diet won't influence the cholesterol level in her breast milk, it can affect the milk's fatty-acid content. For example, when mothers eat a diet rich in polyunsaturated fats like vegetable and corn oil, their milk content of linoleic acid can almost double. Dr. Margot Mellies found this change in the fatty-acid composition of breast milk when she studied fourteen breastfeeding mothers and their infants in the late 1970s. Linoleic acid is an essential fatty acid that is particularly important to the growth and development of infants. So the type of fat we eat can affect the fats in breast milk even though it doesn't affect the milk's cholesterol content.

The current recommendation for adults is that we eat no more than 300 milligrams of cholesterol per day and that our fat intake not exceed 30 percent of our total calories, with not more than 10 percent of that fat from saturated fats. These same prudent guidelines apply to nursing mothers. The meal plan in chapter 6 meets these goals. You'll benefit from following these prudent guidelines while breastfeeding and from continuing them for the rest of your life.

Mothers who have dangerously high cholesterol levels should consult a registered dietitian for specific counseling. Mothers who must follow a low-cholesterol diet while breastfeeding can switch to 1-percent milk, eat only low-fat cheese, trim fat from meats, avoid fried foods, and eat lots of fruits, vegetables, and grains without gobs of butter or rich sauces. Mothers don't need to eliminate eggs, meat, or milk entirely to control cholesterol.

SOMETHING FISHY

Fish-oil supplements, which are rich in the essential fatty acid docosahexaenoic acid, or DHA, have for sometime been popular among individuals who want to reduce their risk of heart disease. The oil is thought to reduce the risk of heart disease by lowering triglyceride levels and reducing the tendency of the blood to clot. Eskimos who eat fish as a dietary staple have much less heart disease than most other people.

In the mid-1980s, Dr. William Harris asked eight breastfeeding mothers to participate in a study of fish-oil supplements. This study was designed to see if by increasing their dietary intake of DHA, mothers could also increase the level of DHA in their breast milk. DHA is abundant in the human brain and eye. Your baby incorporates DHA into her nerve tissues while in the womb and during the first year of her life.

The eight mothers took fish-oil supplements rich in DHA for up to twenty-eight days. The supplements were equivalent to eating 10 to 23 ounces of cod or sole or 3 ounces of salmon or mackerel daily. All the mothers significantly increased the levels of DHA in their breast milk. Their babies were getting more DHA, which could have a positive effect on their eye and brain development.

Should Mothers Take Fish-Oil Supplements?

If you want the health benefits of fish, the best way to get them is from eating fish, not taking capsules. Not much is known about the long-term safety of fish-oil supplements. Eskimos may have less heart disease than other people, but they have a greater incidence of stroke, perhaps because of the oils' effect on blood clotting. Fish-oil supplements can also contain dangerously high levels of vitamins A and D, and they can interfere with the way vitamin E performs in the body. For these reasons, mothers should eat fish, not fish-oil capsules, to get the health-promoting benefits of these fatty acids.

VEGETARIAN DIETS

Some vegetarians simply avoid red meat like beef, lamb, and pork, while others eliminate all animal foods from their diets. It is only at the very strict end of the spectrum when all meat, milk, poultry, and eggs are eliminated that vegetarian mothers and babies risk deficiency.

Cases of malnutrition in breastfed babies have occurred when vegetarian mothers eat extremely restricted diets. In one case, a six-month-old infant was admitted to the University of California Medical Center in San Diego in a coma. He was born apparently healthy to a mother who had consumed no vitamin B_{12} foods such as meat, eggs, or milk for eight years before her pregnancy. The mother had no symptoms of B_{12} deficiency, and her breastfed baby appeared to develop normally until about four months of age, at which time his development started to regress; he became lethargic, irritable, and bruised easily. It is important to note that this little baby had a B_{12} deficiency even though his mother was symptom free. I'm happy to report that the baby improved dramatically within just four days of treatment with B_{12} and was discharged from the hospital after fourteen days, with a prescription for a daily vitamin B_{12} supplement in his mom's hand.

This is an extreme case. Most vegetarian mothers are knowledgeable and careful about what they eat and aware that vitamin B_{12} and vitamin D are crucial to their babies' health. It is only those mothers who are very strict vegetarians who must be cautioned about extreme B_{12} deficiency.

Parents who are vegetarian often want to raise a vegetarian child. This can be safe if the child's diet is planned carefully. A vegetarian child is at much greater risk for nutritional inadequacies than a vegetarian adult. The reason for this is that babies and young children need lots of calories and nutrients. A diet high in vegetables and grains is very bulky and can fill a child up before he has met his protein, calorie, and vitamin needs. An egg provides 70 calories, lots of protein, and many nutrients in one ounce of digestible food. To get the same amount of protein, your child would have to eat one to two cups of rice and beans. You can see the problem.

If you want to plan a vegetarian diet for your child, request a free copy of Teddy Bears and Bean Sprouts (see the Resources section for ordering information).

NURSING YOUR PREMATURE BABY

Babies who come early can definitely benefit from their mothers' breast milk. With support from the medical staff and from their families, mothers with premature babies can successfully nurse their infants.

Mothers of premature babies often have to wait before they can be united with their little ones. Sometimes this separation may be brief, and if the child is strong and can suck, he may be able to nurse quite soon after he is born. But many mothers are separated from their infants for an extended period and must spend their first days and sometimes weeks using a breast pump. This takes tremendous commitment, but nursing your baby, even if it means pumping and storing breast milk, will be tremendously rewarding. Your baby gets the benefit of your healthful breast milk, and you'll get to feel that you're really participating in your baby's care.

Mothers who have premature babies produce preterm milk that is richer in protein, sodium, and chloride, than the milk of mothers with full-term babies. These extra nutrients are essential to meeting a preemie's needs.

Make sure to let your doctor know that you want to breastfeed. A lactation consultant can be a tremendous help to the mother of a premature baby. Your doctor may be affiliated with a lactation consultant; if not, check the Resources section for suggestions on finding a consultant in your area. Check the Resources section too if you need help finding a breast pump.

If you are discharged from the hospital before your baby, try to rest and eat well. This will keep up your milk production and help you maintain your own health. If you must be at the hospital for long periods, bring some good, healthy snacks and ask if there is a spot where you can sit down and put your feet up between feedings. This is a stressful time for you and your family, so pay extra attention to taking good care of yourself.

Good Snacks to Bring to the Hospital

Yogurt in individual containers
Peanut butter and crackers
Juice boxes or cans
Sliced cheese and bread
Whole, ready-to-eat fruit like peaches, pears, and apples

FEEDING THE MOTHER OF TWINS OR TRIPLETS

Common sense alone is going to tell you that the mother of twins or triplets is going to need more food than the mother of a single child. Your body will secrete 420 to 700 calories a day for each child who is being exclusively breastfed, which means that you need an extra 500 calories for each baby being nursed. The good news is that your breasts can meet this demand. Studies show that while most babies drink only 500 to 700 grams of milk daily, a mother can make 2,000 to 3,000 grams if the demand is there. Some mothers supplement breastfeeding with bottle feeding when twins or triplets arrive. They put one child to the breast while the others feed from bottles; at the next feeding, they rotate babies. Mothers who do this are really only nursing one child at a time and need to increase their caloric intake by only 500 calories a day.

TANDEM NURSING

Mothers who conceive before the first nursing child is weaned and then go on to tandem nurse have special needs. The demand for all the nutrients will increase because the mother needs enough nutrition to nourish her pregnancy and to keep up an adequate supply of breast milk without depleting her own reserves. There have been no nutritional studies that identify particular problems of tandem nursing, but these mothers should plan to get the special nutrients needed for lactation (calcium and zinc) plus those needed for a healthy pregnancy (iron, folic acid, and protein). The mom who is tandem nursing doesn't have much room for junk food.

Once the new baby is born, the mother's milk returns first to colostrum and then to the early postpartum milk. The younger infant should nurse first and feed until satisfied. (Usually older children nurse for comfort, not nutrition.) The older child can nurse after the baby is done.

DIABETES AND BREASTFEEDING

Today more and more mothers who have diabetes are delivering happy, healthy babies, and these mothers are being encouraged to breastfeed. Diabetes is greatly affected by diet. A breastfeeding mother who has diabetes must eat a balanced diet that is divided into many small meals. These frequent small meals help keep her blood sugar stable.

There are several types of diabetes: gestational, insulin dependent, and non–insulin dependent. Mothers who developed gestational diabetes while pregnant probably found that it disappeared after they gave birth. The rise in your blood sugar was caused by the stress your baby caused while growing in your womb. After you delivered, your blood sugar probably returned to normal, and your breast milk will not be affected. Women who develop gestational diabetes have an increased incidence of non–insulin dependent diabetes when they get older. In fact, 50 to 60 percent of women with gestational diabetes develop permanent diabetes within five to twenty years. Most women who develop permanent diabetes are overweight and over twenty-five years old. If you had gestational diabetes, you can reduce your risk of permanent diabetes or delay its development by keeping your weight in the ideal range and by exercising regularly.

Mothers with insulin dependent and non–insulin dependent diabetes will want to pay careful attention to what they eat. The information given here is only a guideline. Every mother with diabetes should consult a registered dietitian for specific nutrition recommendations that are coordinated with her physician's care plan. Women with diabetes walk a tightrope. The goal is to prevent high blood sugar while avoiding low blood sugar. It is not uncommon for mothers who take insulin (the hormone that regulates blood sugar) to find that the amount they need decreases while they breastfeed. That's because some of the sugar that would normally circulate in the mother's blood is now being used to make up part of her milk supply. These mothers will need less insulin, and their blood-sugar levels will be lower.

Very low blood sugar, or hypoglycemia, is of course undesirable. Its symptoms include weakness, dizziness, headaches, and possibly even blackouts. Hypoglycemia can inhibit your milk production. To prevent hypoglycemia eat meals at prescribed times, eat more if you exercise, and always carry a quick-acting carbohydrate like sugar packets or glucose tablets. Some nursing diabetic mothers find that they need to decrease their evening dose of insulin to prevent hypoglycemia.

A sample meal schedule for a diabetic mother on 2,700 calories a day might look like this:

| Meal | Portion of the day's allotment | |
	Percentage	Calories
Breakfast—8:00 A.M.	10%	270
Snack—10:00 A.M.	7.5%	202
Lunch—12:00 noon	30%	810

	Portion of the day's allotment	
Meal	Percentage	Calories
Snack—3:00 P.M.	5%	135
Dinner—5:30 P.M.	30%	810
Snack—7:00 P.M.	5%	135
Bedtime snack—10:00 P.M.	7.5%	203
Snack—3:00 A.M.	5%	135

To determine calories, the recommendations given in chapter 6 can also be used by the mother with diabetes. The diet and calorie plan that I use is actually adapted from the exchange system devised by the American Diabetes Association and American Dietetic Association. Many mothers with diabetes will find it familiar.

What is extremely important is when you eat. A mother who has diabetes and who takes insulin should not go for more than three hours without something to eat. If she does, she risks developing low blood sugar. If you find you overeat by consuming half your recommended calories in one sitting, your blood sugar may rise too high. A gentle walk may help lower your sugar level. While breastfeeding, lactose (milk sugar) may be passed in your urine. This means that testing urine for sugar could show you are spilling sugar when you really aren't. Therefore, breast-feeding mothers should use a home blood test to monitor their blood-sugar control.

The diabetic mother needs to get about 20 percent of her calories from protein, 40 to 60 percent from carbohydrates, and 30 to 40 percent from fat. Each snack should include a small amount of protein. In most cases, protein takes longer to digest and can help carry you from meal to meal.

Mothers with diabetes who chose to breastfeed will be happy to learn that breastfeeding may protect their babies from developing the disease. The breast milk of a diabetic mother has been found to be comparable to the milk of nondiabetic moms; the major difference is that the breast milk of diabetics is generally higher in milk sugar. In my research I found no evidence that this was harmful to the baby.

Because diabetes increases the risk of body infection, breast-feeding moms with diabetes must not ignore sore, cracked nipples or signs of mastitis. Call your health-care provider if you suspect any type of infection in your breasts.

One of the greatest obstacles for mothers with diabetes is that frequently their newborns can't be put to the breast immediately after delivery. It is quite possible that your baby will need to be given a physical, have blood drawn, or even need some medical attention. While these procedures are important, they do delay the time until the two of you can be together. The sooner the baby is put to the breast, the more likely the mother and baby will be successful at breastfeeding. Before you deliver, tell your doctor that you want to breastfeed. If she expects a long delay before you can nurse your child, ask if you can use a breast pump in the interim to stimulate your milk production.

IRON-DEFICIENCY ANEMIA

Approximately 15 percent of women of childbearing age have iron-deficiency anemia. Iron is part of the hemoglobin in your blood, which carries oxygen to your cells. Iron-deficiency anemia occurs when your body's stores of iron are depleted. Symptoms include fatigue, weakness, shortness of breath, and pallor. Your iron stores won't be depleted if you skip a meal or don't eat iron-rich foods for a day or two. In most cases, it takes a long time to deplete iron stores. Women are at greater risk for iron deficiency than men because menstruation causes monthly loss of blood and iron. During pregnancy, a woman's blood volume increases, and her developing placenta and baby require iron too, which can further deplete the mother's stores.

The RDA for iron for pregnant women is set at 30 milligrams. For breastfeeding mothers, it drops down to 15 milligrams.

Breastfeeding doesn't draw much iron; a mother secretes less than 1 milligram of iron in a day's supply of breast milk. Less iron is needed while breastfeeding than when you have your period. Since in many cases your period won't resume for several months while you nurse, breastfeeding actually gives you an opportunity to conserve iron, and it's a good idea for women who are iron deficient. But if your period starts again while you are breastfeeding, your demand for iron will increase, so make sure you get some very good sources.

Iron can be a tough nutrient to get, particularly for women on calorie-restricted diets or women who don't eat animal foods like beef, lamb, and so on, which are the best iron sources. The iron that is available from vegetables is less absorbable than the iron in meat. Milk is also a very poor source of iron.

If iron deficiency is a problem for you, try to eat iron-rich foods (a complete listing of these foods is given in chapter 3). There are other things you can try to enhance iron absorption:

- Eat a food rich in vitamin C with every meal—it will enhance absorption of the iron you eat. Drink orange juice, eat a citrus fruit for dessert, or eat a vitamin C–rich vegetable such as tomatoes or broccoli.
- Eat a small amount of meat with every meal.
- Eat iron-fortified cereals, bread, and pasta.
- Cook in cast-iron pots. Studies show that some of the iron passes from the pot into your food and can become a significant source of iron.
- Studies have found that tea and coffee can inhibit iron absorption, so drink these an hour before or after you eat your meal.
- Ask your doctor for an iron supplement. Unfortunately, the iron consumed in tablet form isn't nearly as well absorbed as that from real food. Iron supplements can also be constipating and upsetting to the stomach.

Even if you have iron-deficiency anemia, your baby won't be affected while you breastfeed. Iron-deficiency anemia is quite uncommon in breastfed babies under six months old. Your little one was born with his own six-month supply of iron, even if your intake of iron while pregnant was less than ideal, and this supply helps insure adequate iron levels. The exception to this rule has been seen in breastfed babies who are given solid food early—say at the three-month mark. Early solids can decrease a baby's intake of breast milk, which contains a small but highly absorbable form of iron. Babies who start on solid foods early should get a good iron-rich food. Iron-fortified cereal can be a good choice.

A child who at nine months is still consuming only breast milk can also become iron deficient, because at this age breast milk can no longer supply all her demands for iron. After six months, all breastfed babies need an external iron source. Iron-fortified cereal is a good choice for them too.

HIGH BLOOD PRESSURE

High blood pressure gives no early warning signs. Untreated, it can cause headaches, kidney disease, even stroke. If you've had high blood pressure, make sure you get regular follow-up care. Routine blood pressure readings are the only way to know if you have the disease under control.

Women with high blood pressure can breastfeed. Women who are on medications will need to discuss the fact that they are breastfeeding with their doctors. You may want to talk with both the doctor who is prescribing your medication and your baby's pediatrician. Breastfeeding may actually lower a woman's blood pressure. It serves as a diuretic, pulling extra fluid into the breast milk. The higher levels of prolactin that are present in breast-feeding women may also help lower blood pressure. You may be concerned about what to eat to control your high blood pressure while you breastfeed, but you should meet your needs for feeding the baby first. You'll be glad to hear that the same diet that is healthy for breastfeeding moms can also help control high blood pressure.

Many people are aware that salt has been linked with high blood pressure in some individuals. In these cases, reducing sodium intake can lower blood pressure. Breastfeeding moms can cut back on salt by simply putting away the salt shaker and avoiding foods that are obviously salty.

There is no RDA for sodium, but the minimum adult requirement has been set at 500 milligrams per day. While breastfeeding, a mother's need increases by about 135 milligrams a day, bringing the safe minimum requirement for sodium to approximately 635 milligrams. Since studies have found that the standard American diet provides 1,800 to 5,000 milligrams of sodium a day, you can see that obtaining the 635 milligrams isn't likely to be a problem. By not adding salt to food while cooking or at the table and by avoiding obviously salty foods, you can reduce sodium intake to 2,000 to 4,000 milligrams a day. This generously meets the minimum suggested requirement.

Controlling salt is not the only dietary measure that can help you to manage high blood pressure. Calcium, potassium, magnesium, and alcohol can all have an effect on hypertension.

- Calcium—Calcium has been found to have an antihypertensive effect in some individuals. Make sure you get the RDA.
- Potassium—This mineral may lower blood pressure by depleting sodium. Good food sources of potassium include all fresh fruits and vegetables. Moms should get at least two or three servings of each daily. Fresh meat and poultry are good sources, too.
- Magnesium—Individuals with high blood pressure were able to lower blood pressure by increasing magnesium intake, according to one research study. Breastfeeding moms are encouraged to get adequate magnesium from food, including green leafy vegetables, whole grains, nuts, meat, and beans.
- Calories—Reaching and maintaining ideal body weight can be extremely effective for controlling high blood pressure. A 5-

percent weight loss alone has been found to lower blood pressure and in some cases eliminate the need for medication.

• Alcohol—One percent of American women have high blood pressure because of the amount of alcohol they drink. Women who choose to breastfeed want to follow the recommended restrictions on alcohol to prevent this from being a problem.

Please note that supplements above the RDA are not recommended for any of these nutrients. Food is your best source for them all.

HEMORRHOIDS AND CONSTIPATION

If you have the misfortune of developing these two conditions together, you're going to be uncomfortable. Constipation is technically defined as not having a bowel movement for three days. (In case you didn't know, you don't have to have a daily bowel movement.) If constipation is a problem, look at what you're eating. Foods rich in fiber like fruit, vegetables, whole grain bread and cereals are your friends. (If your diet has been low in fiber, start high-fiber foods slowly; too much all at once might make you uncomfortable.) Raisins, prunes, and figs can be helpful too. Fluids help keep stools soft and prevent constipation, so remember to drink plenty of fluids—the recommendation is two quarts daily while you're breastfeeding.

Most doctors won't recommend a laxative except on a temporary basis. Regular use can become habit-forming, eventually making a bowel movement without a laxative impossible. If constipation is a problem, allow yourself the time to go to the bathroom. That advice might have sounded ridiculous before you had a baby, but as a new mom you might be able to see the problem. Many moms are too busy to allow themselves a few personal moments, and for them constipation can become quite a problem.

If you developed or aggravated hemorrhoids while pregnant,

you're not alone. Because of the increased pressure on the anal opening, lots of pregnant women develop hemorrhoids. Hemorrhoids usually aren't dangerous, but they can become a painful problem if you're constipated, so try to avoid constipation by eating lots of fiber-rich foods. If you have painful hemorrhoids, consult your doctor about medical treatment.

High-fiber Foods

Cereals: All-Bran, Bran Buds, 100% Bran flakes, unprocessed raw bran, Shredded Wheat.

Whole Grains: Brown rice, cracked wheat, bulgur, kasha.

Bread: 100% whole wheat products (sliced bread, pita bread, bagels, English muffins), bran bread, rye bread, Bran'nola pumpernickel. (Always check labels if you're looking for whole grains. The first ingredient should say *whole* wheat. Wheat flour can mean white flour, and this isn't high in fiber.)

Crackers: Any cracker listing whole wheat as the first ingredient, graham crackers, Ry-Krisp.

Beans and peas: Lentils, kidney beans, chick-peas, baked beans.

Seeds and nuts: Sesame, sunflower, pumpkin, and poppy seeds, peanuts with skins, almonds with skins, walnuts, cashews.

Fruit: Apples, grapefruit, grapes, berries, mangoes, melons, oranges, pears, and peaches. Wash well or buy organic and leave the peel on.

Vegetables: All kinds. Wash well and peel waxed cucumbers and peppers.

MOM GOES BACK TO WORK

Rejoining the work force is not a health issue like diabetes or high blood pressure, but it does present unique problems for the nursing mother. Without planning or support by family, friends, employers, and coworkers, a new mother can easily become overwhelmed and overstressed.

Mothers who work outside the home are more likely than others to choose breastfeeding at first, but they are apt to wean sooner or add supplemental bottles. Surveys show that fatigue, difficulty with pumping and milk storage, concerns about adequate milk production, having enough time for work and even enough time to eat are a mother's top concerns when she goes back to her job.

In a study on the working mother and breastfeeding published in the *Journal of Public Health Policy*, six barriers to continued breastfeeding were identified:

1. Lack of good childcare near or at the mother's work site.
2. No place for a mother to nurse, pump, or store milk.
3. Inadequate employment policies regarding maternity leave and job security.
4. Disapproving attitudes regarding breastfeeding by employers and coworkers.
5. Lack of knowledge about breastfeeding on the mother's part.
6. Lack of knowledge about breastfeeding on the part of health-care workers, particularly those involved with employee health.

Being well informed about the hurdles you may face when returning to work is probably your best defense against problems. To make your transition easier, try the following.

- Before you deliver, try to seek out other mothers at your work site to see how they coped.
- Find another mother—a friend, a coworker, or a La Leche League member—to give you firsthand practical advice and support. Lactation consultants can also be real lifesavers.
- Ask your family for help. Having people run errands, prepare some casseroles, or perhaps pick up your baby at the sitter's may make your life easier.

- Consider working part-time or trying to do some work at home. Some lucky moms can job-share, with two people working half of the same job, allowing more time for each to be at home.
- Try to find a childcare situation that's close to work so you can feed your baby during breaks.

While you cope with working and caring for a new baby, remember that breastfeeding doesn't go on forever. When your baby is very little it may seem as though the situation is hopeless and overwhelming. It may give you comfort to remember that it's all temporary. Soon enough—and it may even seem like it's too soon—your baby won't be completely dependent on just you.

GOOD FOODS FOR BUSY MOMS

Eating well while working can be a real challenge. A working mother has to take care of her baby (a full-time job in itself) in addition to her job and household responsibilities. Lots of women put their baby first and leave little time for their own needs. Eating well is important for you *and* the baby. If you don't eat enough, you'll feel even more fatigued and run down.

The best foods are the ones you make from scratch, but I would rather see a mother eat a frozen dinner than skip a meal. Here is a list of healthy ready-to-eat foods that might work for you when you're rushed at work:

- Yogurt
- Ready-made sandwiches from the deli or supermarket
- Frozen dinners (if you have a microwave at work)
- Crackers and a jar of peanut butter (you can keep these in your desk)
- Fresh fruit—apples, bananas, pears
- Nuts

- Dried fruits
- Individual packs of applesauce, fruits, or pudding

There are several good books for mothers who plan to return to work. You can find these listed under "Working Moms" in the Resources section.

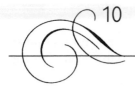

10

EAT WELL, FEEL WELL

MOST OF YOUR USUAL RECIPES CAN BE PART OF YOUR MENU WHILE you're breastfeeding. Some women feel that certain spices, seasonings, or vegetables bother the baby. This is a very individual matter. If you feel some of my ingredients are too strong, just cut back on the amounts I suggest.

You'll be an unusual new mother if you have the time or the desire to do a lot of cooking. But you must feed yourself, and if you make healthy, satisfying foods you'll feel better and so will your baby. Make double portions of recipes and use your freezer to keep ready-to-eat foods on hand.

A NEW DAY IN THE KITCHEN

For many families, a child brings renewed interest in healthy eating. It's not uncommon for people to become more responsible about what they eat once they become parents. Breastfeeding mothers in particular are very conscientious about what they eat. Here's a list of cooking tips that will help your whole family eat healthier:

- Try reducing the fat content in your favorite recipe by half. For example, if you make a chicken stew that calls for four tablespoons of olive oil, simply reduce it to two. No one will notice the difference. (In most cases you can't reduce the fat in baked goods without altering the recipe.)
- Try using water or cooking wine to "sauté" in instead of butter or oil.
- If you're using convenience foods like boxed macaroni and cheese or rice mixes, cut the amount of butter or margarine called for in the directions by one-half.
- Use skim or 1-percent milk in any recipe calling for milk.
- Buy and use low-fat cheeses or substitute for high-fat hard cheeses with smaller amounts of a strong-flavored cheese like Romano or Parmesan.
- Use canned evaporated skim milk to replace cream in recipes such as cream soups.
- Try substituting low-fat yogurt for sour cream in recipes. This can work in baked goods such as coffee cake as well as in a stroganoff dish (keep in mind that yogurt can become a bit runny in a sautéed dish).
- If a recipe calls for a half-cup of vegetables, try doubling that amount to increase your vegetable intake.
- Mix low-fat yogurt with mayonnaise in such things as potato or macaroni salad or when preparing tuna salad. This also works great on green salads—top a large tossed salad with one tablespoon creamy dressing mixed with two tablespoons low-fat plain yogurt.
- Trim all visible fat from meats and bake or broil instead of fry. Regular hamburger can be as low in fat as the more expensive lean choices, depending on how you cook it. If you use it in a meat loaf and the fat is kept trapped in the pan, then it will be high in fat. If you broil a hamburger on a pan that allows the

fat to drip away, then it will be just as low in fat as the lean burger.

- Trim the skin from poultry.
- When making soups or gravies, refrigerate and later remove the fat that rises to the surface.
- Sprinkle confectioners' sugar on cake instead of high-fat frosting.
- Cooking can destroy nutrients. To get the most out of the food you buy, try the following:

  Keep ripe fruits and vegetables cold.

  Cook vegetables for as short a time as possible and with as little water as possible.

  Don't pare or trim vegetables excessively—the leaves on broccoli stems, for instance, are very nutritious. Do peel waxed produce. Don't wash or soak vegetables for prolonged periods.

  Avoid boiling vegetables.

START YOUR DAY OFF RIGHT

A good breakfast is essential to maintaining your energy, especially while you're breastfeeding. Even if you weren't a breakfast eater in the past, you should feel hungrier now and should want to eat breakfast. You don't have to eat eggs and sausage. A morning meal of fruit, cereal with milk or yogurt, toast, juice, and a cup of coffee will give you protein, calcium, and carbohydrates and a good start on your day's nutrients.

A good breakfast should provide 20 to 25 percent of your calories (that's about 540 to 675 calories). Many mothers will feel better if they include some protein at breakfast to carry them through the morning. This might be cheese, milk, peanut butter, yogurt, cooked fish, eggs, ham, or beans.

TEN NO-FUSS BREAKFAST IDEAS

Some of these meals can be put together the night before. Our house is always busy in the morning, so having food ready to heat helps reduce the morning frazzles.

1. Cereal with milk and fruit.
2. Baked eggs. (Mix 2 eggs with 1 tablespoon of milk and, if you wish, 1 tablespoon grated cheese and 2 tablespoons chopped tomato. Put together the night before. Bake at 375° F for fifteen minutes or until firm, or microwave for two minutes on high, stir and cook one minute more, and let rest one minute covered before serving.
3. Oatmeal with milk and fruit. Mix ¼ cup oatmeal with ¼ cup milk plus ¼ cup water and let stand overnight. Cook per instructions in the microwave or on the stove, then top with fresh fruit.
4. Grandma's Early Morning Coffee Cake with a dish of yogurt and fresh fruit (see page 173 for recipe).
5. Frozen waffles topped with yogurt and fresh fruit.
6. Poached egg on an English muffin.
7. Bagel topped with cottage cheese, sliced tomato, red onion, and black pepper (the onion and pepper are optional). The sliced tomato is an excellent source of vitamin C.
8. Breakfast fruit shake. Put 1 cup yogurt and 1 cup canned or fresh fruit (seeded and peeled) in the blender the night before. Mix in the morning. Enjoy a few toasted slices of good bread along with it.
9. Mini hamburger. Cook a ground-beef patty instead of sausage or bacon. Serve with sliced tomato, whole-wheat toast, milk, and a slice of fruit. At $1.79 a pound, ground beef is a much better protein buy than bacon or sausage, which is also often higher in fat.
10. Peanut butter on whole-wheat toast with sliced bananas.

Start Your Day with Zinc

While you're nursing, you need to eat about 16 to 19 milligrams of zinc every day. A cereal rich in zinc is a great way to help meet that requirement. The zinc content of selected cereals is listed below. Not all the zinc you eat in food will actually get absorbed, which makes it extra important for you to select zinc-rich foods.

Cereal	Zinc in 1-cup serving (mg)
All-Bran	11.1
Apple Jacks	3.7
Bran Buds	11.1
Cap'n Crunch	4.01
Nutri-Grain cereals (all varieties)	more than 5.3
100% Bran	5.74
Special K	2.77
wheat germ	18.9*

* Great source of zinc, but it contains 432 calories and 12 grams of fat.

RECIPES FOR HEALTHY EATING

Now that you know good nutrition is important while breastfeeding here are some recipes that combine good taste with good nutrition. I have tried to keep the preparation time very short and the ingredient lists short. To help you use the menu-planning system from chapter 6, I've included the number of portions from each food group that the recipes provide.

HOME-BAKED BREAKFASTS

Eating a good breakfast is the best way to start your day. Whole grain cereal, fresh fruit, and milk or yogurt is a simple and nutritious start. When you feel like baking and have the time, try one of the recipes that follow.

GRANDMA'S EARLY MORNING COFFEE CAKE

When I was a little girl my mother would occasionally treat her brood of four hungry children to this special coffee cake. She assembled it the night before, refrigerated it, then added the topping and baked it while our family got dressed and ready for school. She made it again when she came to help me out when my girls were born, and it brought back fond memories of warm family breakfasts. I hope you enjoy it!

Cake
3 tablespoons butter
½ cup sugar
1 egg, beaten
1 cup milk
1 teaspoon vanilla extract
1½ cups flour
1 tablespoon baking powder
¼ teaspoon salt
⅔ cup wheat germ

Topping
2 tablespoons wheat germ
3 tablespoons sugar
3 tablespoons melted butter
¾ teaspoon cinnamon
5 tablespoons crushed corn flakes

Preheat the oven to 375° F. Cream butter with sugar. Add egg, milk, and vanilla extract, then add dry ingredients and blend well. Grease an 8-inch square or round cake pan. Pour batter into pan. Mix topping ingredients together and sprinkle over batter. Bake for 25 to 30 minutes, or until it tests done with a cake tester.

TO MAKE AHEAD: Mix cake, pour into pan, mix topping, but do not sprinkle on cake. Refrigerate covered. Before baking, add topping.

Makes nine portions; 1 starch and 1 fat exchange per serving.

WHOLE-WHEAT AND BRAN MUFFINS

These muffins taste good and provide lots of fiber and zinc. Of course they're easy to make, too.

¾ cup wheat bran
¾ cup whole-wheat flour
½ cup Bran Buds
½ cup brown sugar
2 teaspoons baking soda
¼ teaspoon salt
2 teaspoons grated orange or
    lemon peel (use organic or
    unwaxed fruit)

1 egg, lightly beaten
⅔ cup plain yogurt
¼ cup vegetable oil

Preheat the oven to 400° F. Mix all dry ingredients, including grated peel. In a separate large bowl, mix the egg, yogurt, and oil and blend well. Fold in dry ingredients until just blended—don't overbeat. The batter will be thick and grainy looking. Pour into lightly oiled muffin tins and bake for 18 to 20 minutes.

Makes twelve muffins; 1 starch and 1 fat exchange per muffin.

VARIATIONS: To make blueberry or raisin muffins, fold in 1 cup of blueberries or ½ cup of raisins to the finished batter and cook as directed.

MAIN DISH WINNERS

The recipes that follow are designed to be low in fat, high in flavor. Ingredients should be readily available in your market and the recipes easy to assemble. Enjoy!

CREAMY PASTA PRIMAVERA

Years ago when my husband and I decided to eat less fat, we developed this recipe for a rich, creamy pasta. When I became a new mother, I really liked this recipe because it was fast, healthy, and a great way to get more calcium.

1 pound pasta
1 clove garlic, chopped
1 tablespoon olive oil
2 carrots, scrubbed and diced
1 cup fresh or frozen green vegetables (broccoli, peas, green beans, zucchini)

1 cup plain low-fat yogurt
1 cup low-fat cottage cheese
2 tablespoons grated Parmesan cheese

Bring a large pot of water to boil for the pasta. In a large frying pan, sauté the garlic in oil; add the raw carrots (and raw green vegetables if you're using them). Cover and let simmer on the lowest heat about 5 minutes, then remove from heat. If using a frozen green vegetable add it in the last minute of cooking. Vegetables should be tender but not mushy.

Add the pasta to the boiling water and cook according to the package directions. Meanwhile, blend the yogurt, cottage cheese, and Parmesan cheese in a blender until creamy and smooth. Drain pasta. Toss with the yogurt-cheese sauce and three-quarters of the cooked vegetables. Arrange on serving dish and sprinkle with remaining vegetables. Serve hot with extra grated cheese, bread, and a good salad.

This makes four good-size portions; 4 starch, ¼ milk, 1 fat, 1 protein, and 1½ vegetable exchanges per serving.

YOGURT-FRIED CHICKEN

Fried chicken went off our menu years ago, but I miss the crispy texture. This recipe is a terrific way to get the taste of fried food and lots of protein and calcium without all the fat. If you shy away from cooking with yogurt, try this at least once. It does not have a sour yogurt taste.

8 chicken thighs (use another cut if you prefer)
2 cups plain yogurt
1 cup seasoned bread crumbs
2 teaspoons olive oil

Preheat oven to 375° F. Remove skin from chicken, roll in yogurt, coating chicken liberally. Then roll in seasoned bread crumbs. Place on a lightly oiled baking dish. Drizzle with the olive oil and bake for 45 minutes.

This recipe makes four portions; 1 starch, ½ milk, and 4 protein exchanges per serving.

PASTA WITH FISH SAUCE

Lots of people don't eat fish because they think it smells or don't know how to cook it. Please try this dish even if you aren't a fish lover. It's easy and oh so good!

1 pound cut-up white fish such as cod, haddock, halibut, or pollock (frozen will do but thaw first)
½ cup white wine
½ cup water
1 tablespoon fresh chopped parsley
¼ teaspoon dried thyme
Juice from ½ lemon
1 clove garlic, chopped
2 tablespoons olive oil
1 pound pasta

In a medium-size saucepan, combine the fish with the wine, water, parsley, and thyme. Bring to a boil and reduce heat to a simmer and cook for 10 minutes. Fish should be hot and flaky; don't overcook. Add the lemon juice. Remove from heat.

Sauté the garlic in olive oil. Cook pasta, drain, and pour into a bowl. Pour in all of the fish and its cooking liquid plus the sautéed garlic. Toss. Serve while hot.

Makes four portions; 2 starch, 1 fat, and 4 protein exchanges per serving.

SALMON CROQUETTES

If you select canned salmon with the bones still in, you'll be eating a superb calcium source. Many people object to the texture of the bones. You can reduce this complaint by mashing and chopping the salmon when the recipe calls for mixing. This makes twelve croquettes. If you don't eat them all at one meal, simply freeze them.

1 can salmon, drained
*   (14¾-ounce size)*
1 cup dried bread crumbs
¼ cup low-calorie
*   mayonnaise*
½ cup finely chopped onion
½ cup finely chopped green
*   pepper*

1 egg
1 teaspoon good prepared
*   mustard*
1 teaspoon Worcestershire
*   sauce*

Preheat the oven to 350° F. Mix all the ingredients, reserving ½ cup of bread crumbs. Mix until all ingredients are well blended. Shape into twelve cone-shaped croquettes. Roll croquettes in the remaining bread crumbs. Bake on a slightly greased cookie sheet for 15 minutes. Serve topped with Yogurt Dill Sauce.

Makes four three-croquette portions; 1 starch, 1 fat, and 4 protein exchanges per serving.

YOGURT DILL SAUCE: Mix 1 cup plain yogurt, 2 teaspoons dried dill or 1 tablespoon fresh minced dill, and 2 teaspoons lemon peel chopped fine or grated (buy a pesticide-free or unwaxed lemon).

Makes four ¼-cup servings; ¼ milk exchange per serving.

ONE MORE FISH DISH

Eighty percent of American kitchens now have microwave ovens, and fish cooks beautifully in the microwave. When I make this dish I like to buy a small portion of two or three different types of fish. For instance, I might have 5 ounces each of shark, marlin, and salmon. It's a great way to vary the recipe and to compare the flavors of the various fish.

> 1 pound fish steak (tuna, swordfish, salmon, marlin, shark) or any combination that equals 1 pound
> 6 tablespoons good olive oil
>
> 2 tablespoons fresh lemon juice
> 1 teaspoon Dijon mustard
> 1 tablespoon chopped fresh dill, parsley, or chives

Cut fish into 2-inch cubes. Arrange on a 9-inch microwave-safe glass pie plate. Cover with a microwave-safe glass plate. Cook on high power for 3 minutes.* Remove cover carefully; it will be hot. Rotate the fish so that any undercooked fish is moved to the outside of the dish. Cook 1 minute more, covered, on high power.

Mix remaining ingredients together. Pour over fish and let rest for 2 or 3 minutes to finish cooking. I like to serve this over hot pasta or cooked rice.

Makes four portions; 1 fat and 4 protein exchanges per serving.

*The cooking times are given for a 700-watt microwave with a carousel unit. Small ovens may require longer cooking times.

BROWN RICE AND BROCCOLI

I absolutely love brown rice cooked with wheat berries. It gives a gourmet touch without any fuss at all. My supermarket doesn't carry wheat berries, so I buy them in a specialty food shop or the health-food store.

1 clove garlic, or 1 small
  onion, chopped
1 tablespoon olive oil
1 cup brown rice
½ cup wheat berries
3 cups boiling water
½ teaspoon salt (optional)

3 cups broccoli, chopped
  (1 large head)
1 pound tofu, cubed
1 tablespoon soy sauce
3 ounces cheddar cheese,
  grated

Sauté the garlic (or onion) in oil in a heavy 10-inch skillet for 1 minute. Add the rice and wheat berries, cook 1 minute, and stir. Add the boiling water and salt. Bring to a boil, stir, and cook for 30 minutes, covered, on low heat.

Add chopped broccoli and cook 5 minutes more, or until broccoli is tender. If the rice looks dry, add another ¼ cup of water when the broccoli is added (you don't want the rice to dry out or it will burn). Toss in tofu and soy sauce. Mix all ingredients, sprinkle with grated cheese, and cover. Remove from heat and let rest for 2 or 3 minutes, or until cheese melts.

Makes three portions; 2 starch, 1 fat, 2 vegetable, and 3 protein exchanges as per serving.

BEAUTIFUL BEAN AND VEGGIE SALAD

This is easy but very pretty and delicious. I developed it one day when I had to get something on the table fast and only had leftovers to work with. It was a hit!

1 can kidney beans, rinsed
10 black olives, sliced
1½ cups cooked corkscrew
  noodles (rotini)

1½ cups cooked chopped
  broccoli
2 tablespoons low-calorie
  Italian dressing

Mix all ingredients together. Serve warm or refrigerate for 1 hour.

Makes three portions; 1 vegetable, and 2 starch exchanges per serving.

CURRIED CHICKEN

This is a great way to use up leftover chicken or turkey. If you think you don't like curry, try this recipe, but put in only the amount of curry you think you can handle. If you refuse to eat curry, substitute an equal amount of dried dill.

1½ cups cubed chicken	¾ cup plain yogurt
(about 12 ounces)	1 tablespoon curry powder
1 tablespoon mayonnaise	½ cup sliced red grapes

Toss cubed chicken with mayonnaise and yogurt. Sprinkle with curry, fold until well blended. Stir in grapes. Serve on lettuce or in pita bread.

Makes three portions; ¼ milk, 1 fat, 1 fruit, and 3 protein exchanges per serving.

QUICK-COOKING CHILI

1 pound ground beef or	1½ cups canned crushed
ground turkey	tomatoes
½ onion, chopped	1 tablespoon chili powder, or
2 cups kidney beans	½ package of taco
(a 16-ounce can)	seasoning mix
2 cups corn (fresh or frozen)	salt (optional)

Sauté ground beef in a large saucepan on medium heat for 5 minutes. Drain off fat. Add onion, sauté 2 to 3 minutes more. Add beans, corn, tomatoes, chili powder or taco seasoning. Simmer for 10 minutes. Taste and add more chili powder or salt if desired.

Makes five portions; 2 starch, 1 fat, 2 vegetable, and 3 protein exchanges per serving.

BROCCOLI SALAD

Keep a batch of this in your refrigerator. It's a tasty, easy way to get healthy veggies.

*1 ½ cups broccoli cut into
  1-inch pieces
½ cup carrot chunks (cut
  carrot in half lengthwise
  then into 1-inch chunks)*

*2 tablespoons Italian
  dressing*

Steam vegetables for 5 minutes. If you have a microwave, you can sprinkle with water and microwave covered in a microwave-safe dish for 3 minutes at full power, then stir and cook 1 minute more.

Put cooked vegetables in a bowl and toss with salad dressing. Serve warm or chilled.

Makes two 1-cup portions; 1 fat and 2 vegetable exchanges per serving. Use low-calorie dressing and reduce the fat by half.

QUICK SPAGHETTI SAUCE

Because of the added vegetables, this is more like a ratatouille than a conventional spaghetti sauce. Serve it over your favorite pasta.

*1 pound ground beef
  or turkey
2 cups tomato puree or
  crushed whole tomatoes*

*1 cup any combination
  of chopped zucchini,
  mushrooms, and green
  peppers
1 teaspoon oregano*

Sauté the ground beef in a saucepan for 5 minutes on medium heat. Drain the fat and add the tomatoes, vegetables, and oregano. Bring to a boil, then simmer on low for 2 minutes.

Makes four 1-cup portions; 1 vegetable and 4 protein exchanges per serving.

VEGETABLE MEAT LOAF

This is a great way to get some extra veggies. The vegetables add flavor as well as nutrients to the meat loaf.

1 pound lean ground beef or ground turkey

2 cups finely grated vegetables, any combination: carrots, zucchini, mushrooms, green beans, green peppers, onion

1 cup crushed crackers, unsweetened flake cereal, or bread crumbs

salt and pepper

1 egg

Preheat oven to 350° F. Mix all ingredients in a bowl until they are all well blended. Clean hands work best for mixing. Press into a 8-inch by 4-inch loaf pan. Bake for 50 minutes or until done. After 20 minutes of cooking pour off accumulated grease and continue cooking.

Makes four portions; 1 starch, 1 vegetable, and 4 protein exchanges per serving.

VEGETABLE STEW

Here's an easy recipe that can use any green you have available. Green leafy vegetables are a great way to get extra calcium.

1 clove garlic, chopped

1 tablespoon olive oil

1 pound chopped greens (spinach, kale, turnip greens, or any combination)

4 cups chicken or vegetable broth

¼ pound thin spaghetti broken into 1-inch pieces

1 pound firm tofu cut into 1-inch cubes (optional)

Gently cook the garlic in the oil over low heat until tender. Do not brown. Add the well-washed chopped greens and mix. Cover and cook over low heat for 5 minutes. Add the broth, bring to a boil, and add the pieces of raw pasta. Reduce heat to low, cover, and simmer for 20 minutes. If you're adding tofu, stir it in after 15 minutes of cooking and let it simmer with the vegetables for the remaining 5 minutes.

Serve in bowls with good crusty bread, some grated cheese, and even a splash of soy sauce.

Makes four good-size portions; 1 starch, 1 fat, and 1 vegetable exchange per serving. If you add tofu, count it as 1 protein exchange per serving.

HUNTER'S PIE

This is a variation of shepherd's pie, only easier because you don't need to mash the potatoes. I also use either fresh or frozen peas and corn, depending on what's available. They will cook or thaw once in the oven.

*1 pound ground beef
or ground turkey
2 tablespoons chili sauce
1 cup peas, fresh or frozen
1 cup corn, fresh or frozen*

*4 small potatoes, sliced thin
4 teaspoons margarine,
melted
salt and pepper (optional)*

Preheat the oven to 350° F. Lightly oil a microwave- and oven-safe 1-quart casserole dish. Cook the ground beef for 3 minutes on high power in the microwave. Drain the fat, mash the lumps, and mix in the chili sauce. Some of the meat will still be red. Layer the corn and peas over the meat, then arrange the sliced potatoes in a circular pattern on top of the vegetables. Drizzle the margarine on top of the potatoes, sprinkle with salt and pepper if desired, and bake for 40 minutes, until potatoes are tender.

Makes four portions; 2 starch, 1 fat, and 4 protein exchanges per serving.

MEALS IN A BLENDER

Busy new mothers may find it helpful to keep ready-to-drink nutritious shakes on hand in the refrigerator. When I was home with Sarah and too busy to make a snack, I relied on these. I made a batch in the morning and sipped on it through the day. It was something I could easily handle while I nursed my new daughter.

BANANA FRAPPÉ

1 cup low-fat milk   1 ripe banana
½ cup orange juice

Mix all ingredients in a blender. Serve in a tall glass or over ice.
    Makes two large portions; ½ milk and 1 fruit exchange per serving.

ORANGE CREAM

Some mothers just don't like plain milk. Here's a fabulous recipe that contains over 250 milligrams of calcium in one serving.

1 6-ounce can frozen orange   1 teaspoon vanilla extract
    juice   1 cup water
1 cup nonfat dry milk   2½ cups ice cubes

Blend all ingredients in the blender, adding ice cubes gradually.
    Makes three portions; 1 milk and 2 fruit exchanges per serving.

HEALTHY DESSERTS

Desserts can be a part of our meals if we choose those that provide nutrition as well as taste. The choices that follow are low in fat but high in flavor and nutrition.

YOGURT SUNDAE

This isn't exotic, but it looks pretty enough to be a fattening, forbidden food. I make it in a champagne goblet for an elegant presentation.

1 cup good yogurt (plain or vanilla)
½ cup fruit, any type

¼ cup granola or other crunchy cereal

Put one-half the yogurt in the bottom of the dish and top with granola. Layer the remaining yogurt on top with the fresh fruit.

Makes one portion; 1 starch, 1 milk, and 1 fruit exchange per serving.

WHOLE-WHEAT BREAD PUDDING

Here is a way to get fiber, calcium, zinc, and protein all in one dish. What a great way to get nutrition!

2 slices whole-wheat bread, toasted
1 cup milk
1 egg, slightly beaten

2 tablespoons honey, or 1 tablespoon honey and 1 tablespoon molasses or maple syrup

Preheat the oven to 350° F. Tear the toast into 1-inch pieces. Mix all ingredients in a bowl until the bread is well coated. Pour into a lightly greased 4-cup baking dish. Bake for 30 minutes. Serve topped with ½ cup ice milk.

Makes two portions; 1 starch, ½ milk, 1 daily option, and ½ protein exchange per serving.

INDIAN PUDDING

This is one of my absolutely all-time favorites and very easy to make.

1 cup cornmeal   3 tablespoons molasses
2 cups milk

Mix all ingredients in a microwave-safe glass dish. Cook in the microwave for 3 minutes on high power, uncovered. Stir, cook for 2 more minutes. Let rest, covered, for 2 minutes. The pudding should be thick and creamy; if it gets too thick, stir in ¼ to ½ cup more milk.

Makes four portions; 1 starch, ½ milk, and 1 daily option exchange per serving.

BAKED PEARS

These can be prepared in the microwave or in a conventional oven. Topped with yogurt and served with a crisp gingersnap, they are refreshing and wholesome.

1 pear   1 tablespoon brown sugar
½ cup boiling water

Slice pears in half, remove core and stem. Place cut side down on lightly oiled baking dish. Mix together sugar and water, pour over pears.

Microwave oven: Cook on high power, uncovered, for 3 minutes. Cover and let rest for 2 minutes.

Conventional oven: Bake at 350° F, covered, for 20 minutes.

Makes one portion; 1 fruit and 1 daily option exchange per serving.

BLUEBERRY SAUCE

We try to keep the intake of simple sugars low in our house. To use less syrup on pancakes and waffles, we came up with this fabulous creation. When the blueberries cook they release their own juices, making a "syrup."

1 cup fresh or frozen
blueberries

2 tablespoons maple syrup

Combine fruit and syrup in a small saucepan. Cook for 10 minutes on medium heat, covered. Allow to cool. Use as you would maple syrup.

Makes one portion; 1 fruit and 1 daily option exchange per serving.

FAT-FREE CHOCOLATE SYRUP

I love the taste of chocolate. Cocoa powder by itself is almost fat free. This recipe has no added fat and it satisfies my craving for chocolate. Use it to top ice milk or frozen yogurt.

2 tablespoons unsweetened
cocoa
1 to 2 tablespoons sugar

2 tablespoons water (instead
of water you can try a
sweet liqueur like Grand
Marnier and omit half the
sugar)

Mix sugar and cocoa in a small, heavy saucepan. Add liquid and stir over medium-low heat. The powder will eventually absorb the liquid. Heat until the mixture is well combined and some of the liquid evaporates, about 2 minutes. Remove from heat before boiling or it will become too thick.

Makes two portions; 1 daily option exchange per serving. The sugar and cocoa have no redeeming nutritional qualities, so they can't be counted in any of the food groups. Use this just occasionally.

GOOD QUICK CAKE

Here's a simple, tender cake that can be prepared and on the table within 30 minutes. Read the variations below to discover ways to dress it up by adding some special mix-ins. Another super plus is that there is no added fat in this cake—the only fat comes from the eggs.

1½ cups all-purpose flour	¼ teaspoon salt
⅔ cup sugar	1 cup yogurt, plain
2 teaspoons baking powder	2 eggs
½ teaspoon baking soda	

Preheat the oven to 375° F. Mix all the dry ingredients together. In a separate bowl, combine the yogurt and eggs. Mix thoroughly. Fold yogurt mixture into dry ingredients until blended, but do not overmix. Pour into a lightly oiled tube-cake pan or an 8-inch square cake pan. Bake for 20 minutes or until top is golden.

Makes twelve portions; 1 starch exchange per serving.

BLUEBERRY CAKE: Gently fold in ¾ cup fresh or frozen blueberries after all ingredients have been mixed. Bake as directed.

BANANA CAKE: Mix 1 small, very ripe banana (approximately ½ cup) into the yogurt and egg mixture. Mash it in well, fold yogurt mixture into the dry ingredients, and bake as directed.

SOMETHING TO SNACK ON

There are no bad snacks—just bad snack choices! Choose foods that are nutritious and you actually help your body.

Munchies

These are good snacks to keep around for when you've got to have something to eat but don't want to eat high-fat, not-so-good-for-you junk food.

- Air-popped popcorn
- Angel food cake (serve with fruit and low-fat yogurt or ice milk)
- Graham crackers
- Animal crackers
- Hard candy (fat-free candy and gumdrops can help those of you with an urge for sugar. They contain no vitamins or minerals. If they prevent a binge on candy bars, then they can be considered a good snack choice.)
- Gumdrops
- Fruit
- Sliced peppers
- Pretzels
- Rice cakes
- Breadsticks
- Water ice/Popsicles/fruit pops

Stamina Snacks
These snacks have protein to carry you to the next meal.

- Hard-cooked eggs
- Cheese melted on a soft tortilla
- Low-fat cottage cheese on a cracker
- Peanut butter on graham crackers or rice cakes
- Nuts (careful how many you eat—high in fat)
- Soup—choose a broth soup with meat or beans
- Yogurt
- Mini pizza—melted cheese on an English muffin topped with tomato and oregano
- Hummus with pita bread
- Baked potato with a slice of cheese melted on top

BE A SMART SHOPPER

There are a lot of foods at the supermarket or health-food store that are easy to prepare and good for you, too. The lists below give my recommendations for nutritious, low-fat foods. In most cases, the simpler the food, the more nutritious it is. A fresh broccoli stalk is a better nutrition buy than a package of frozen chopped broccoli with cheese sauce.

The emphasis in my selections is to keep fat intake low. This doesn't mean that breastfeeding mothers have unique fat requirements. All of us—new mothers, grandparents, fathers, brothers, and sisters—should be more careful about the amount of fat we put into our bodies.

Reading Labels

Food packages list ingredients with the predominant item first. A sweetened cereal with sugar listed as a first ingredient would be loaded with sugar. A cereal with sugar as the third or fourth ingredient would have a much lower sugar content. Be leery of labels that tout "No Cholesterol" or "99% Fat Free," as these claims can be misleading. For instance, several brands of peanut butter claim they have no cholesterol. The consumer would assume these were better products than the ones that did not carry the low-cholesterol claims. The truth is that no peanut butter contains cholesterol because peanuts are plant foods, and only animal foods contain cholesterol. Words like "fresh" and "all natural" don't carry much meaning either. Your best bet is to read labels carefully and try to choose as many wholesome, unprocessed foods as possible.

When evaluating products for fat, read how many grams of fat are listed on the nutrition label. Each five grams of fat is the equivalent of one pat (one teaspoon) of butter.

Dairy Products

Cheese: Try the low-fat varieties, including the lower fat cottage cheeses and "diet" sliced or American cheese.

Milk: Low-fat milk of all kinds, buttermilk, chocolate skim milk.

Yogurt: Try yogurt with a fat content of only 0 to 3 grams per 8-ounce serving.

Meats

Deli Counter: Chicken or sliced turkey is your best bet. Lean meats like roast beef, turkey ham, turkey pastrami, and lean ham are okay choices. Try to skip the high-fat cold cuts, pastrami, and hot dogs.

Poultry: All chicken and turkey is a good choice; try not to eat the skin. Cornish hens are a good choice, too, but duck is quite high in fat. Ground turkey and chicken can be substituted for ground beef in recipes, helping to lower fat intake.

Red Meat: All lean meats such as steaks and trimmed chops can be good selections. When cooking a stew or soup that calls for ground beef, buy lean or extra-lean beef for that recipe, because the fat will be cooked in. The less expensive higher fat ground beef can be used if the fat can be drained off during cooking. Avoid high-fat meats such as bacon, sausage, short ribs, corned beef, or pastrami. If you do have these meats, keep the portions small.

Fish: All plain, unprocessed fish is a good choice. Don't be afraid to use frozen fish. It's tasty when baked and usually costs less than fresh fish.

Fats

Oils: All vegetable oils are cholesterol free because they are extracted from vegetables. Vegetables carry fats that are thought to be good for us; these are known as polyunsaturated and monounsaturated fats. Oils vary in their composition of polyunsaturated and monounsaturated fats, flavor, and cooking properties. Good choices include canola, corn, olive, safflower, soybean, sunflower, peanut, and sesame oils. Butter and margarine both contain an equal number of calories. Butter contains cholesterol and saturated fats that can raise a person's blood cholesterol. Margarine, however, contains no cholesterol and very small amounts of saturated fat. Lard also contains saturated fat, and shortenings are treated in such a way that much of the fat they contain is also saturated. Remember, all oils contain approximately 45 calories per teaspoon.

Salad Dressings and Mayonnaise: There are so many good low-fat versions and even fat-free products on the supermarket shelf that you shouldn't have much trouble selecting one that tastes good to you. Read labels and select one that supplies less than 5 grams of fat per serving. Remember that these foods give us mostly flavor and not much nutrition.

Fruit

All fresh fruits are good choices. I often treat myself to the more expensive "exotic" fruits like papaya or mango—they seem like more special desserts. Frozen fruits prepared without sugar are good choices, too. Be cautious of dried fruits. They're easy to snack on but carry a lot of calories.

Vegetables

All fresh veggies are great. In fact, I think they make a good quick snack: a half-cup of any vegetable can be chopped and ready to eat after just two minutes of cooking in the microwave. Canned vegetables always contain more salt than fresh varieties unless they are specially marked. Plain frozen vegetables are great, too. Watch out for the vegetables that are frozen with butter or cheese sauces; they're packed with fat calories.

Starches

Bread: Most breads are naturally low in fat and are packed with B vitamins and healthy carbohydrates. Exceptions are cheese breads, butter breads, or rolls. Baked goods such as croissants, muffins, and biscuits are higher in fat than sliced breads. Try to get into the habit of buying whole grain breads. They contain more fiber than white bread and therefore can be a better health choice.

Cereals: These grain foods are a terrific way to get nutrition. When selecting cereal try to buy the whole grain types without added sugar or fat (granola cereals can be quite high in fat). Read labels and buy a cereal that contains 0 to 3 grams of fat per serving.

Pasta and Rice: These are superb foods when purchased in their simple, unadorned state. Convenience pasta and rice packages that require lots of added butter or margarine are not good choices. When I use these convenience foods I always cut the amount of butter suggested by one-half or two-thirds. The ramen-style noodles are very high in fat because they are fried after cooking, then dried and packaged.

Frozen Foods

If you shop smart you can find some healthy foods in the freezer case. Most are ready to serve, which makes them very useful to new mothers. Your best choices are simple foods like the frozen fruits and vegetables. Frozen rice or pasta dishes without sauces are good too (we love the ready-to-cook frozen raviolis and manicottis.). Frozen pizza crust lets you make your own healthy pizza in just minutes. Sprinkle a frozen crust with low-fat cheese, a bit of pureed tomato sauce, and fresh or frozen vegetables and cook at 350° F until the cheese melts and veggies are tender—about ten to fifteen minutes.

Frozen Desserts: Fruit bars, frozen low-fat yogurt, Italian ices, and fudge bars are good selections. Ice milk is good, too. Premium ice creams contain much more fat and should be saved for special treats.

Generally, the more expensive the ice cream, the higher its fat content.

Frozen frosted cakes and pies aren't great choices, but frozen plain cakes can be.

Frozen Entrées: More and more frozen dinners are being slimmed down by their manufacturers, and these can be good quick choices for hurried moms. They all contain more sodium than the same food prepared from scratch. In many cases, the low-calorie frozen dinners may be too low in calories for you. Most supply only 300 to 350 calories; a breastfeeding mother will need closer to 600 calories at a meal. To add the extra low-fat calories you'll need, try eating a couple of slices of good whole-wheat bread with just a bit of butter or margarine spread on.

Frozen burritos are quick meals if you like and can tolerate beans. They contain about 350 calories each, with 30 percent of those calories coming from fat.

Canned Foods

All canned meats, mixed dishes, and vegetables have added salt unless they are specifically marked "no salt added." The only exception to this is canned fruit, which usually has extra sugar. There are good canned foods to choose from, however. I always keep a supply of broth-based canned soups on hand. I know they have more sodium than the ones I make from scratch, but let's face it—I can't always make my own broth. I prefer the broth soups over cream soups because the latter have more fat. I also like canned beans because they are more convenient than soaking and cooking my own. I just rinse the salt off before using. Canned fruits without added sugar are also a good bet. I rarely if ever buy canned mixed dinners because I don't like the taste. However, a canned chili or stew might appeal to you, though it will be higher in sodium and probably lower in protein and vegetables than one you make yourself.

Seasonings

All seasonings, including herbs and spices, are okay to use. Herbs and spices with salt added are best avoided; I recommend unsalted varieties such as onion powder over onion salt. Breastfeeding mothers who feel that some seasonings bother their babies can simply avoid or reduce these seasonings while nursing.

GRANDMA'S BEST BETS

My mother is a superb cook, and she graciously volunteered to stay for a week when Sarah was born and help out her overwhelmed daughter. Not only did she do a magnificent job caring for me, David, and the house, she also left me with a freezer full of delicious meals. She left a sliced cooked pot roast, a batch of great tomato sauce in two-cup portions, and the following recipes, ready to reheat. If your mother comes to visit, ask her to put a few of these in the freezer, too.

CHICKEN IN THE POT

This is a recipe my mother gave me for quick cooking. It never made its way into the freezer—we ate it too fast.

2 cloves garlic	1 bay leaf
3-pound whole chicken	4 carrots, peeled and cut in
4 cups water	chunks
1 onion, peeled	4 stalks celery, chopped
½ teaspoon thyme	4 potatoes, peeled and cut in
3 sprigs parsley	quarters
6 peppercorns	

Place a clove of garlic in each end of chicken. Put chicken in a heavy pot along with neck and gizzards and remaining ingredients. Bring to a boil; cover and simmer for 1 hour. Serve chicken on a platter surrounded by cooked vegetables. Use the stock as a gravy for the potatoes.

Makes about 8 portions; 1 starch, 1 vegetable, and 4 protein exchanges per serving.

HAMBURGER SOUP

This makes a good-size pot; you can eat some and then freeze the rest. It contains protein, vegetables, and starch in one meal. Accompany the soup with a glass of milk and some sliced bread or a salad and you have a healthy, tasty meal. If you allow this to cool in the refrigerator before eating, all the fat rises to the top and can be skimmed off. This trick saves lots of fat calories without harming the taste at all.

2 onions, chopped	1 bay leaf
1 tablespoon margarine or vegetable oil	9 peppercorns
	½ teaspoon thyme
½ to 1 pound lean ground beef	3 ribs celery, chopped
	3 carrots, sliced
2 cans consommé, or 4 cups broth	2 potatoes, diced
	3 tablespoons fresh parsley, chopped
1 large can whole tomatoes	

Sauté onions in the margarine or vegetable oil until tender. Add hamburger and cook 5 minutes. Drain fat. Add consommé plus 3 cans of water or broth. Stir in tomatoes, bay leaf, peppercorns, thyme, chopped celery, sliced carrots, diced potatoes, and parsley. Bring to a boil; quickly reduce to low heat, and simmer for at least 1 hour. Best if made early in the day.

Makes four portions; 1 starch, 1 fat, 2 vegetables, and 2 to 4 protein exchanges per serving.

CHILIBURGER SOUP

You can use either ground beef or ground turkey in this recipe. This soup contains protein, vegetables, and starch from the barley.

2 onions, chopped
1 tablespoon vegetable oil
3 celery stalks, chopped
1 pound ground meat
1 32-ounce can tomato juice

½ teaspoon to 1 tablespoon
    chili powder
½ cup pearl barley,
    uncooked

Sauté onions in oil until tender. Add celery and ground meat and cook for 5 minutes, mashing lumps. Drain fat. Add tomato juice, chili powder, and barley. Bring to a boil, then reduce heat and simmer for 1 hour.

Makes four portions; 1 fat, 2 vegetable, and 4 protein exchanges per serving.

VARIATION: In the last 10 minutes of cooking, add 1 cup of any fresh vegetable: corn, peas, green beans, zucchini. If using frozen vegetables, add in the last 5 minutes of cooking. This will add half of a vegetable exchange.

WHEN FRIENDS ASK, "WHAT CAN I DO?"—TELL THEM!

I received many wonderful gifts from friends and family, but one of the most memorable and timely was from my neighbor Valerie. Sarah wasn't even a week old and it was early afternoon. I heard a knock on the door and opened it to find Valerie standing there with a bag full of food. She had a large salad, a fresh vegetable quiche, a full bottle of wine, and an entire chocolate cake from the bakery. David and I were absolutely thrilled to have a complete meal delivered to the house. We savored every bit and drank small celebratory glasses of wine. I must confess that the chocolate cake went quite quickly.

So when friends ask what can they do, take them up on their generosity and give them some ideas:

- Ask them to make you some home-cooked food like a stew or casserole.
- If you don't feel comfortable with that, ask them to go to the store and buy you some good ready-to-eat foods. A quick trip to the supermarket can yield a fresh roasted chicken, a large salad from the salad bar, and a loaf of good bread.
- If you have older children, ask friends if they could take the kids for a while so you can have some time alone with the new baby.
- If they are really good friends, let them do the laundry or clean the house.
- If they want to help you out with a gift, suggest a certificate for a cleaning service or a diaper service.
- If you need a breast pump when you return to work, maybe they would want to help you out with the cost of renting one. Every mother who has used a top-of-the-line battery-run or electric breast pump has been very impressed with their ease and efficiency. They cost about two to three dollars per day to rent. Look in the Resources section for ordering information.
- My good friend Marilyn gave me a card with a coupon in it to be redeemed for five hours of baby-sitting. I didn't use this until Sarah was about four months old, but it was a wonderful gift and it gave me a sense of independence knowing that I could count on one of my best friends to take care of Sarah when I needed time to myself.

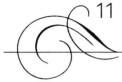

11

QUESTIONS, ANSWERS, AND PROBLEM SOLVING

SOME COMMON CONCERNS

When I first became a mother I kept a daily diary. Most of these questions are taken from the problems and concerns that I wrote down. I think many new mothers also face these issues, so this question-and-answer section was added to help find answers to these common concerns.

How often should I let my baby nurse?
Breastfed babies do best if they can feed on demand. In the beginning, this helps to establish a good milk supply. Your baby will probably want to feed every two to three hours, but some may want to eat every hour at the beginning. Breastfed babies often seem to eat more frequently than bottle-fed babies.

How will I know if my baby is getting enough to eat?
Your baby should wet at least five to eight diapers every day. In the first months, he should have two to five bowel movements

daily (this drops off after the second month). When you bring him for his first weight check at two weeks, he should be gaining weight and growing in length and head circumference. If he also appears happy and content, you can be pretty sure he's getting enough food.

I want to use a breast pump but I can't seem to get the hang of it. What should I do?
The letdown reflex is a complex but natural chain of events. When your baby suckles at your breast, hormones and chemicals in your body are triggered to send milk to your breast and baby. You need to establish the letdown reflex in order to pump successfully. This means relaxing. Find yourself a quiet spot and think about your baby. You can also try applying a warm face-cloth to your breasts or giving yourself a gentle breast massage. Then place the pump over the areola and operate according to its instructions. Many mothers have reported better luck with battery-operated or electric pumps than with manual pumps. If this still doesn't work, hunt out a fellow mom who has successfully pumped or contact the La Leche League or a lactation consultant for support. Most mothers find that with practice, pumping becomes easier.

What is a lactation consultant and how do I find one?
A lactation consultant is an allied-health-care worker with special training in assisting mothers with unusual and routine breastfeeding situations. Such a consultant provides education and consultation and is usually affiliated with a medical team. There are no universal guidelines regarding education or licensing, so ask for credentials.

To find a lactation consultant, ask your doctor or midwife or look in the Resources section at the back of this book. The mothers I have talked with who needed and used a lactation consultant consider them lifesavers. One mother with a premature child said that if it were not for her lactation consultant, she never would have had enough support to nurse her baby boy. Another mother whose baby girl didn't nurse well was referred to a lactation consultant who arranged for the mother to try a special feeding device known as a Lact-Aid Nursing Trainer. The device worked wonders, and mother and baby had a healthy, happy nursing experience.

How can I find a qualified nutritionist?
Ask your health-care provider for the name of a dietitian or nutritionist. If he or she can't recommend one, then look in the yellow pages. It doesn't really matter if they call themselves nutritionists or dietitians, because the word "nutritionist" has no legal definition. Anyone from a vitamin salesman to a doctor can use the term. Do look for a registered dietitian (R.D.). These professionals have attended college and completed advance studies in nutrition, either as interns or in a master's-degree program in nutrition or a related field. They have also passed an extensive exam in nutrition, and they must keep up their registration by completing continuing education courses in nutrition every year.

What should I look for in a nursing bra?
A breastfeeding woman doesn't need to wear a bra if she doesn't want to, but a good nursing bra can give your breasts extra support. For women who wear bras, it can make feeding time easier and more comfortable because the bra flap lifts easily, allowing baby to feed. Select a bra that's all cotton, because cotton breathes better than synthetics and allows extra moisture to evaporate, keeping you more comfortable. Avoid underwire-type nursing bras, because the wires can block milk ducts and cause discomfort. Most women find that while nursing they need a bra that is one to two sizes larger than their prepregnancy bra.

What can I do if my breasts become engorged?
Breast engorgement isn't uncommon and it can be very uncomfortable. To relieve the discomfort, try warm heat such as a hot shower or moist cloth.

If your breast engorges, massage it before feeding the baby; you may also need to manually express some milk to soften the breast so your baby can latch on easier. Allow your baby to nurse at the engorged breast first—this is when he is most hungry and his sucking will help relieve engorgement.

The key to overcoming engorgement is to try and avoid it in the first place; feed early and frequently from birth on.

How can I prevent sore nipples?
Proper positioning of baby at the breast can help, as can allowing your breast to air dry after each feeding. Of course this is a bit tough in public. When you're not at home, try wiping any excess milk off with a clean cloth moistened with plain water.

I'm a thirty-five-year-old mom. Does age affect how much milk I make?
A study of 155 mothers ranging in age from fifteen to thirty-seven years old was conducted and reported in *Human Lactation 2* (Plenum Press, 1986). The researchers studied how much milk these mothers made and its nutritional composition. Milk volume was not related to age. There were some differences in milk fat and lactose content between moms of different ages, but the significance of these findings is unclear. In short, older mothers (and there are many more of us these days) can breastfeed successfully.

If breast milk is the perfect food for baby, why is my pediatrician telling me to give him vitamins?
Breast milk is the perfect food for your baby because it is intensely rich in nutrients. Doctors who suggest supplements are simply trying to provide an extra margin of safety against possible deficiencies of key nutrients. Usually supplements are advised for vitamins D and K, fluoride, and iron for the following reasons:

- Vitamin D: If your baby doesn't get much exposure to sun, a daily supplement of 5 to 7.5 milligrams of vitamin D will be recommended.
- Vitamin K: All babies are given a dose of vitamin K at birth to

protect them against hemorrhaging. Regardless of the type of feeding method chosen for the baby, vitamin K injections are given as a safety measure.

- Fluoride: If the fluoride content of your household water supply is low, then fluoride will be advised because adequate fluoride is thought to reduce your baby's chance of cavities.
- Iron: By the time a child is six months old, he needs to start eating foods rich in iron. If intakes of these foods are low, iron supplements will be recommended.

Most pediatricians do not recommend multivitamins for nursing babies because your breast milk supplies all the calories and nutrients needed (except for the occasional exceptions mentioned above).

My baby is now two months old and I want to lose weight. Can I try Weight Watchers or a liquid diet?
Liquid diets are not recommended for breastfeeding mothers. These regimens usually advise the dieter to take one diet drink at breakfast and one at lunch, then eat a small meal at suppertime. Each diet drink provides only 250 to 300 calories. If supper weighs in at 500 calories, a mother following this diet would be eating less than 1,200 calories a day. At this level, she won't be able to meet her requirement for most nutrients, and her milk production may actually decline. So please, no liquid diets designed for rapid weight loss.

Weight Watchers has a menu designed for both pregnant women and nursing mothers. The Weight Watchers regime is much better than a liquid diet, but it isn't optimal. There may be too few calories for some women, and the recommended number of servings of starch is definitely too low. In most cases, the group leaders of a Weight Watchers program won't be familiar with the recommended safe weight loss for nursing mothers or their unique nutritional needs. If you decide to use the Weight Watchers program, you must assume personal responsibility for getting enough food and losing weight slowly and safely.

Is it safe to take diet pills sold without a prescription?
No. Drugstore diet pills contain high levels of caffeine (as much as 200 to 280 milligrams in a day's dose). This is equivalent to drinking two to three extra cups of coffee per day. If these pills are consumed regularly, enough caffeine could accumulate in your breast milk to be harmful to your baby.

My doctor says that breastfed babies don't grow as fast as formula-fed babies. He seems to be encouraging me to add formula. Do breastfed babies need formula?
Your doctor is right. After the first two to three months, breastfed babies usually do gain weight at a slower rate, but this may be normal. Rate of weight gain is an important indicator of health, but it's not the only factor, and slow weight gain alone doesn't mean the child is failing to thrive. Dr. Ruth Lawrence, in her book *Breastfeeding: A Guide for the Medical Profession,* suggests that a child who is slow to gain weight but "alert, bright and responsive" should be classified as a slow gainer. A child who is not gaining weight, is apathetic, has a weak cry and poor skin tone, wets very few diapers, and passes few stools may be a true case of failure to thrive. Dr. Lawrence's book would be a good book to recommend to any physician needing more information on the development of the breastfeeding baby. While slow weight gain alone doesn't necessitate the use of supplemental formula, if your baby has any of the symptoms of failure to thrive, you need to work with your doctor to meet your baby's nutritional needs.

I work in a city maternity ward, and some of my mothers are infected with HIV, the AIDS virus. Should they be encouraged to breastfeed?
Studies show that 30 to 40 percent of the babies born to mothers infected with the HIV virus will test positively for the infection

themselves. Whether an HIV-positive mother should be encouraged to breastfeed her baby in hopes of transmitting health benefits is unclear. In the United States, the Centers for Disease Control has advised mothers who test positive for HIV not to breastfeed. The World Health Organization in 1987, and again in 1991, recommended that breastfeeding be encouraged especially in developing countries because breastfeeding has known health benefits and the risk associated with transmitting the HIV virus via breastmilk is not known. As you can see, more research needs to be done before we'll have an answer to your question.

WEIGHT LOSS STRATEGIES AND BEHAVIOR MODIFICATION

Knowing what is good and healthy to eat is not all we need to help us eat better or lose weight. The way our families react to diet changes or altered exercise programs can make a big difference in our success in meeting our goals. If you feel you have problems that interfere with your ambitions for changing eating habits, you aren't alone. Most of us find that lack of time, our families' eating preferences, and the foods that friends drop off as gifts get in the way of our intended goals. And old eating habits die hard. The problems that follow may sound familiar to you. You'll be interested to see how you can turn them around to your advantage.

My husband works late, so I feed the children at five o'clock and eat with them. Even though I have already eaten, I'm hungry again when my husband gets home, and I pick enough to make up another meal. How can I stop eating the equivalent of two meals each night?
Eat your full meal at five o'clock and eat a planned snack later. A salad or some cooked vegetables or an appropriate snack such as a yogurt sundae could be enjoyed with your husband.

When friends drop by, they either bring something to munch on or I pull something out of the freezer. Most of the time I end up overeating. What can I do?

Talk with your friends. Tell them that you want to eat healthier and ask them to help you out. Foods such as fruits and vegetables would be appropriate munchies. A tray of sliced fresh fruits sprinkled with lemon can be terrific. Or serve simple low-fat crackers, breadsticks, or pretzels with some really good tangy mustard for dipping. Chances are your friends will enjoy the healthier change, too.

I eat out at restaurants quite a bit and feel that I can't manage what I eat. Any suggestions?

Restaurants can actually be helpful to anyone trying to eat healthier. You can't automatically go back for seconds, and you can control what is brought to the table. Do the obvious: select baked or broiled foods, order a salad, request that extra rolls and butter be removed from the table. Ask to split dessert with your dinner partner, or have a bowl of good fresh fruit instead of a calorie-laden cake or pie.

I'm hungry all the time. How can I satisfy my hunger without over-eating?

If you're hungry all the time, then you're probably not eating enough, or you aren't sitting down and taking enough time to enjoy a full meal. New mothers are often pressed for time, and lunch may be a half of a sandwich crammed in while you do the laundry. This kind of eating doesn't provide you with enough food or the satisfaction associated with eating a relaxed, pleasurable meal. Start taking the time to eat three meals a day plus snacks. Allow at least fifteen minutes for a meal.

If you're eating as much as you should based on my guidelines and you're still hungry, munch on low-fat snacks. See page 189 for some ideas. If you're eating enough and still losing weight faster than recommended for nursing mothers, you may need to talk to your doctor. Unsatisfied hunger can indicate medical problems.

I live with my mother, and she cooks too much. If I don't eat everything she makes, she gets mad at me. What can I do?

This can be a hard problem for someone trying to eat differently. The person doing the cooking often uses food to express affection. If you refuse the food, it can be interpreted as a rejection of that person. Ask your mother for her help. Tell her she's a great cook but that since you've had the baby you're trying to eat a little differently: more fruits and vegetables, fewer fried foods, and only the amounts you feel you need. Then tell her the foods you want to stay away from and whatever other changes you plan to initiate, such as no second portions or no added gravy. Then stick to what you say. If one day you say you won't do this and the next day you do, she'll get a mixed message and you'll be right back where you started.

I keep cookies and chips around for my older children. How do I stop picking on them myself?

If you can't control yourself around snack foods that aren't very healthful, the only solution is to stop bringing them into the house. Tell your children about the change. Instead of keeping high-calorie snack foods around, make them special-occasion treats. You can take everybody out for a treat once a week or make a special coffee cake, a great homemade cake, or buy a specialty bakery cake. Freeze any leftovers so you won't be tempted to nibble. The point here is to not have ready-to-eat snack foods around that you can't resist.

My stepchildren visit on weekends and I always feel I have to make big fancy meals. How can I do this and watch what I eat?

First of all, you're probably going to be too tired to make big fancy meals once your new baby arrives. Your stepchildren need to have good, healthy food, but they don't need fancy or elaborate meals. The same foods that are good for you are good for your family. Meals should have at least two vegetables, a main dish, some starch, and perhaps some fruit for dessert. Try any of the ideas in the recipe section, or adapt your old family favorites using my healthier eating guidelines in chapter 10.

I'm a single mother and cooking for one is just too much. How can I get healthy meals?

When your baby is still on breast milk alone, it's hard to prepare big meals just for yourself. If this is your problem, try some of my ready-to-eat suggestions in chapter 10. Not eating good food is not an option for you.

SIX EATING STRATEGIES

Here are some simple eating strategies that can help you stick to your healthy new diet while you breastfeed—and, I hope, for all the years while you watch your new baby grow up.

1. Don't skip meals.
2. Try to eat in one place or eat only if sitting down (this helps me not pick at food while I cook).
3. Don't keep troublesome foods in the house. Stock up on snacks that are good for you: popcorn, breadsticks, and fruit. Keep sliced vegetables on hand.
4. Ask your family, friends, or partner for help in eating better.
5. Incorporate healthy exercise into your life.
6. Chew your food well and eat slowly. This is a good habit, and if you do it, your kids are more likely to do it, too.

AN INVITATION TO MY READERS

It's always exciting to hear from the people who read my books. If you have any comments about the information in this book or want to share a personal experience, I'd like to hear from you.

Write to me, Eileen Behan, at Villard Books, 201 East 50th Street, New York, NY 10022.

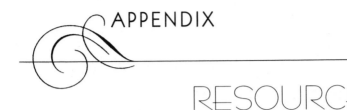

APPENDIX

RESOURCES

ORGANIZATIONS THAT MAY BE OF HELP TO NEW MOMS

Allergies
If you have questions about allergies, contact the following group for more information:

Asthma and Allergy Foundation of America
1835 K Street, N.W., Suite T 900
Washington, DC 20006
(202) 293-2950

Breast Pumps
I called each of the 800 numbers below, and all were manned by courteous, helpful operators. When you call, the operator will tell you where you can rent the breast pump of your choice. If

you have questions about the use of a pump, contact the La Leche League for support or find a lactation consultant.

The three top manufacturers of electric or battery-operated pumps:

Medela: 1-800-435-8316
Ameda/Egnell: 1-800-323-8750
White River: 1-800-824-6351

Diabetes

Most doctors have lots of free information pamphlets about diabetes, the diabetic diet, and diabetes medications. If you need more help, contact the American Diabetes Association:

American Diabetes Association
149 Madison Avenue
New York, NY 10016
212-725-4925

Exercise Guides for New Moms

Anderson, Bob. *Stretching.* Bolinas, Calif.: Shelter Publications, 1980.

Postnatal Exercise Program. This is a video endorsed by the American College of Obstetricians and Gynecologists. Cost: $39.95. To order call 1-800-423-0102 or write:

ACOG Home Health Series
EDN/Saddle River Marketing
Route 727 West
P.O. Box 45
Bridgewater, VA 22812

Lactaid

To obtain more information about Lactaid, which can make milk more digestible for lactose-intolerant people, write or call the manufacturer:

Lactaid
McNeil Consumer Products
P.O. Box 85
Camp Hill Road
Fort Washington, PA 19034
1-800-LACTAID

Lactation Consultants and Organizations

If you have questions about breastfeeding and need some additional professional help, contact these organizations:

International Lactation Consultant Association
201 Brown Avenue
Evanston, IL 60202
708-260-8874

The Lactation Institute
16161 Ventura Boulevard
Suite 223
Encino, CA 91436
818-995-1913
(in Long Beach, California, 213-630-7136)

La Leche League International
P.O. Box 1209
Franklin Park, IL 60131
(708) 455-7730 or 1-800-LALECHE

The La Leche League is made up of experienced breastfeeding moms who volunteer their time and experience to help new mothers. Accredited La Leche League leaders will in most cases have the same skill levels as lactation consultants—plus valuable firsthand experience. You can usually find the number of your local La Leche League group in your phone book.

Nutritionists

To find a registered dietitian, look in the yellow pages under Nutritionist or Dietitian; choose a professional who is a registered dietitian (R.D.). You can also call or write the association below for information about registered dietitians in your area:

American Dietetics Association
216 West Jackson Boulevard, Suite 800
Chicago, IL 60606-6995
1-800-877-1600

Pesticides

For more information about pesticides and children, contact the Natural Resource Defense Council. A booklet called *For Our Kids' Sake* can be purchased from the council. It is published by Mothers and Others for Pesticide Limits and offers practical advice on limiting your child's exposure to pesticides.

Natural Resource Defense Council
40 West Twentieth Street
New York, NY 10011
212-727-2700

HELPFUL PUBLICATIONS

Eating Safely

A new release by the publishers of the health newsletter *Nutrition Action Letter* is *Safe Food: Eating Wisely in a Risky World* by Michael Jacobson, Lisa Lefferts, and Anne Witte Garland. This practical book takes the sensationalism out of this issue and gives you enough useful information to let you make sound, reasonable food decisions.

Safe Food
Center for Science in the Public Interest
1875 Connecticut Avenue, N.W., Suite 300
Washington, DC 20009-5728
202-332-9110
$9.95

Vegetarian Diets

Teddy Bears and Bean Sprouts is a free twenty-four-page booklet on planning and preparing a vegetarian menu for children. You can order it by calling 1-800-4-GERBER.

Other good books on vegetarian cooking:

Lappe, Frances Moore. *Diet for a Small Planet.* New York: Ballantine Books, 1971. This is a very good resource for anyone wanting to learn more about planning a balanced, healthy vegetarian menu.

Robertson, Laurel, Carol Flinders, and Brownwen Godfrey. *Laurel's Kitchen.* New York: Bantam, 1978. A handbook for vegetarian cookery and nutrition.

Working Moms

There are several good books for mothers who want to learn how other mothers handled the transition back to work:

Brazelton, T. Berry. *Working and Caring.* Reading, Mass.: Addison-Wesley, 1985.

Grams, Marilyn. *Breastfeeding Success for Working Mothers.* Sheridan, Wy.: Achievement Press, 1985.

Olds, Sally Wendkos. *The Working Parents' Survival Guide.* New York: Bantam Books, 1983.

Great Nutrition Resources

The following newsletters offer good, timely, and accurate nutrition information in a very readable form:

Nutrition Action Health Letter
Center for Science in the Public Interest
1875 Connecticut Avenue, N.W., Suite 300
Washington, DC 20009-5728
202-332-9110
$19.95 for twelve issues

Tufts University Diet and Nutrition Letter
New Subscription Information
P.O. Box 57857
Boulder, CO 80322-7857
1-800-274-7511
$20.00 for twelve issues

The University of California Wellness Letter
P.O. Box 420148
Palm Coast, FL 32142
$20.00 for twelve issues

Here are some good books on nutrition, feeding kids, and healthy eating:

Behan, Eileen. *Microwave Cooking for Your Baby and Child.* New York: Villard Books, 1991.

Brody, Jane. *Jane Brody's Good Food Book: Living the High Carbohydrate Way.* New York: Bantam, 1985.

Brody, Jane. *Jane Brody's Nutrition Book: A Lifetime Guide to Good Eating for Better Health and Weight Control.* New York: W. W. Norton, 1985.

Connor, William, and Sandra Connor. *The New American Diet.* New York: Simon & Schuster, 1986.

General Breastfeeding Books

The Womanly Art of Breastfeeding. Franklin Park, Ill.: La Leche League International, 1981.

Eiger, Marvin, and Sally Wendkos Olds. *The Complete Book of Breastfeeding.* New York: Workman Publishing Co., 1981.

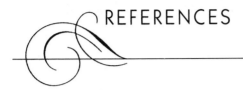# REFERENCES

Much of the nutrition and health research included in this book was based on the 1991 report *Nutrition During Lactation* written by the Subcommittee of Nutrition During Lactation of the National Academy of Sciences in Washington, D.C. Nutritive data was obtained from *Nutritive Value of American Foods in Common Units*, Agricultural Handbook No. 456 (U.S. Department of Agriculture, Washington, D.C., 1975) and *Understanding Nutrition* (St. Paul, Minn.: West Publishing Company, 1990). The bibliography that follows lists the references for additional research used in each chapter.

Chapter 1

Elias, Marjorie F., et al. "Sleep/Wake Patterns of Breastfed Infants the First Two Years of Life." *Pediatrics* 77, no. 3 (March 1986): 322–29.

"Seven of Ten Women for Breastfeeding." *Medical Tribune*, November 1986.

Chapman, Judy J., et al. "Concerns of Breastfeeding Mothers from Birth to 4 Months." *Nursing Research* 34, no. 6 (1985): 374–77.

"To Nurse? The Black and White Picture." *Science News*, March 26, 1988, 203.

Howie, Peter W., et al. "Protective Effect of Breastfeeding Against Infection." *British Medical Journal* 300 (January 6, 1990): 11–16.

Bauchner, Howard, J. M. Leventhal, and E. D. Shapiro. "Studies of Breast-feeding and Infections: How Good Is the Evidence?" *Journal of the American Medical Association* 256, no. 7 (August 15, 1986): 887–92.

U.S. Department of Commerce, Bureau of the Census. *Statistical Abstract of the U.S.,* 385, chart 637. U.S. Department of Commerce, Washington, D.C., 1991.

Martinez, G. A., and F. W. Krieger. "Milk Feeding Pattern in the U.S." *Pediatrics* 75, no. 6 (December 1985): 1004–8.

Ross Marketing Research. *Incidence of Breastfeeding 1951–1987.* August 1987.

Labbok, Miriam. "Does Breastfeeding Protect Against Malocclusion?" *American Journal of Preventive Medicine* 3 (July–August 1987): 227–32.

Chapter 2

Committee on Nutrition, American Academy of Pediatrics. "Nutrition and Lactation." *Pediatrics* 68, no. 3 (September 1981): 435–43.

Hopkinson, Judy M., and N. F. Butte. "Maternal Nutrition During Lactation." *Nutrition and the M.D.* 13 (February 1987): 1–3.

Bachrach, S., J. Fisher, and J. S. Parks. "An Outbreak of Vitamin D Deficiency Rickets in a Susceptible Population." *Pediatrics* 64, no. 6 (December 1974): 871–77.

Sims, Laura S. "Dietary Status of Lactating Women." *Journal of the American Dietetic Association* 73 (August 1978): 139–46.

"Complementary Feeding for Breastfed Infants." *Nutrition and the M.D.* 15, no. 3 (March 3, 1989): 3.

Thomas, M. R., et al. "The Effects of Vitamin C, Vitamin B_6, Vitamin B_{12}, Folic Acid, Riboflavin, and Thiamin on the Breastmilk and Maternal Status of Well Nourished Women at 6 Months Postpartum." *American Journal of Clinical Nutrition* 33 (October 1980): 2151–56.

Chapter 3

Bolton, R.A. "Fluoride Supplementation of the Breastfed Infant." *Journal of the American Medical Association* 263, no. 16 (April 25, 1990): 2179.

Higginbottom, M. C., L. Sweetman, and W. L. Nyhan. "A Syndrome of Methylmalonic Aciduria, Homocystinuria, Megaloblastic Anemia and Neurologic Abnormalities in a Vitamin B_{12} Deficient Breastfed Infant of a Strict Vegetarian." *New England Journal of Medicine* 299, no. 7 (August 17, 1978): 317–23.

Chan, G. M., et al. "Effects of Increased Calcium Intake Upon the Calcium and Bone Mineral Status of Lactating Adolescent and Adult Women." *American Journal of Clinical Nutrition* 46 (1987): 319–23.

Bachrach, Fisher, and Parks. "Outbreak of Vitamin D Deficiency Rickets." 871–77.

Anderson, D. M., and W. B. Pittard. "Vitamin E and C Concentration in Human Milk with Maternal Megadosing." *Journal of the American Dietetic Association* 85 (1985): 715–17.

Salmenperä, L. "Vitamin C Nutrition During Prolonged Lactation: Optimal in Infants While Marginal in Some Mothers." *American Journal of Clinical Nutrition* 40 (November 1984): 1050–56.

West, K. D., and A. Kirksey. "Influence of Vitamin B_6 Intake on the Content of the Vitamin in Human Milk." *American Journal of Clinical Nutrition* 29 (September 1976): 961–69.

Chapter 4

Dusdieker, P. J., et al. "Prolonged Maternal Fluid Supplementation in Breastfeeding." *Pediatrics* 86 (1990): 737–40.

Stumbo, P. J., et al. "Water Intakes of Lactating Women." *American Journal of Clinical Nutrition* 42 (November 1985): 870–76.

Chinese American Food Practices, Customs, and Holidays. The American Dietetic Association, Chicago, Ill., and the American Diabetes Association, Alexandria, Va., 1990.

Mexican American Food Practices, Customs, and Holidays. The American Dietetic Association, Chicago, Ill., and the American Diabetes Association, Alexandria, Va., 1989.

Chapter 5

Kaitschuck, G. K. "Breastfeeding and Losing Weight." *American Baby,* May 1991, 32.

Manson, JoAnn, et al. "A Prospective Study of Obesity and Risk of Coronary Heart Disease in Women." *New England Journal of Medicine* 322 (March 29, 1990): 882–89.

Illingworth, P. J., et al. "Diminution in Energy Expenditure During Lactation." *British Medical Journal* 291 (February 15, 1985): 437–41.

"Diminution in Energy Expenditure During Lactation," letter to the editor and author's reply. *British Medical Journal* 292 (April 12, 1986): 1016–17.

Blackburn, M. W., and D. H. Calloway. "Energy Expenditure and Consumption of Mature, Pregnant and Lactating Women." *Journal of the American Diatetic Association* 69 (July 1976): 29–37.

Butte, N. F., et al. "Effect of Maternal Diet and Body Composition on Lactational Performance." *American Journal of Clinical Nutrition* 39 (February 1984): 296–306.

Ohlin, A., and S. Rossner. "Development of Body Weight During and After Pregnancy." In *Obesity in Europe 88: Proceedings of the First European Congress on Obesity.* Stockholm, Sweden: John Libby and Co., 1989.

"Energy Intake and Lactation Performance in Women." *Nutrition Reviews* 45, no. 1 (January 1987): 12–14.

Strode, M. A., et al. "Effects of Short-term Calorie Restriction on Lactational Performance of Well Nourished Women." *Acta Paediate* 75 (1986): 222–29.

Brewer, Marie M., M. Bates, and L. Vannoy. "Postpartum Changes in Maternal Weight and Body Fat Deposits in Lactating vs. Nonlactating Women." *American Journal of Clinical Nutrition* 49 (1989): 259–65.

Manning-Dalton, C., and L. H. Allen. "The Effect of Lactation on Energy and Protein Composition, Postpartum Weight Change and Body Composition of Well Nourished North American Women." *Nutrition Research* 3 (1983): 293–308.

Whichelow, M. "Success and Failure of Breastfeeding in Relation to Energy Intake." *Proceedings of the Nutrition Society* 35 (1976): 62A–63A.

Chapter 7

American College of Obstetricians and Gynecologists. *Exercise During Pregnancy and the Postnatal Period.* Washington, D.C.: American College of Obstetricians and Gynecologists, May 1985.

American College of Obstetricians and Gynecologists. *Safety Guidlines for Women Who Exercise.* Washington, D.C.: American College of Obstetricians and Gynecologists, May 1986.

Lovelady, Cheryl A., B. Lonnerdal, and K. G. Dewey. "Lactation Performance of Exercising Women." *American Journal of Clinical Nutrition* 52 (1990): 103–9.

Schelkon, P. H. "Exercise and Breastfeeding Mothers." *The Physician and Sportsmedicine* 19, no. 4 (April 1991): 109–16.

American College of Obstetricians and Gynecologists. *Women and Exercise.* Washington, D.C.: American College of Obstetrics and Gynecology, June 1989.

"Baby Jogger Guidelines," letter to the editor. *The Physician and Sportsmedicine* 19, no. 2 (February 1991): 34.

Pacelli, L. C. "Parent-Infant Workouts: More Harm Than Help?" *The Physician and Sportsmedicine* 18, no. 6 (June 1990): 135–43.

Chapter 8

Mennella, J. A., and G. K. Beauchamp. "Maternal Diet Alters the Sensory Qualities of Human Milk and the Nursling's Behavior." *Pediatrics* 88, no. 4 (October 1, 1991): 737–44.

Rogan, W. J., et al. Polychlorinated Biphenyls and Dichlorodiphenyl Dichloroethene in Human Milk: Effects on Growth, Morbidity and Duration of Lactation." *American Journal of Public Health* 77 (1987): 1294–97.

"Infant Dioxin Exposures Reported High." *Science News*, April 26, 1986, 264.

Resman, B. H., H. P. Blumenthal, and W. J. Jusko. "Breastmilk Distribution of Theobromine from Chocolate." *The Journal of Pediatrics* 91, no. 3 (1977): 477–80.

Tyrala, E. E., and W. E. Dodson. "Caffeine Secretion into Breastmilk." *Archives of Disease in Childhood* 54 (1979): 787–800.

Lawrence, Ruth. *Breastfeeding: A Guide for the Medical Profession.* St. Louis: C. V. Mosby, 1989.

Little, R. E., et al. "Maternal Alcohol Use During Breastfeeding and Infant Mental and Motor Development at One Year." *New England Journal of Medicine* 321 (1989): 425–30.

Mennella, J. A., and G. K. Beauchamp." The Transfer of Alcohol to Human Milk." *New England Journal of Medicine* 325 (October 3, 1991): 981–85.

U.S. Department of Health and Human Services. "Lead in Wine." September 9, 1991. Press release.

Munoz, L. M., et al. "Coffee Consumption as a Factor in Iron Deficiency Anemia Among Pregnant Women and Their Infants in Costa Rica." *American Journal of Clinical Nutrition* 48 (1988): 645–51.

Chapter 9

Heggen, L., and R. Becker. "Gestational Diabetes." *Diabetes Forecast Magazine*, 1984. Reprint published and made available by the American Diabetes Association, New York, N.Y.

Datta, T. "Breastfeeding in Cesarean Babies." *Indian Pediatrics* 27 (1990): 86–87.

Butte, N. F., et al. "Milk Composition of Insulin Dependent Diabetic

Women." *Journal of Pediatric Gastroenterology and Nutrition* 6 (1987): 936–41.

Jakobsson, I., and T. Lindberg. "Cow's Milk as a Cause of Infantile Colic in Breastfed Infants." *The Lancet*, August 26, 1978, 437–39.

Chandra, R. K. "Maternal Dietary Engineering Reduces the Incidence of Allergic Eczema." *Breastfeeding Abstracts* 7, no. 7 (Summer 1987): 1.

Jakobsson, I., and T. Lindberg. "Cow's Milk Proteins Cause Infantile Colic in Breastfed Infants." *Pediatrics* 71, no. 2 (February 1983): 268.

Clyne, P. S., and A. Kulczycki. "Human Breast Milk Contains Bovine IgG; Relationship to Infant Colic?" *Pediatrics* 87, no. 4 (April 1991): 439–44.

Knopp, R. H., et al. "Effect of Postpartum Lactation on Lipoproteins, Lipids and Apoproteins." *Journal of Clinical Endocrinology and Metabolism* 60 (March 1985): 542–47.

Harris, W., E. Connor, and S. Lindsey. "Will Dietary Omega-3 Fatty Acids Change the Composition of Human Milk?" *American Journal of Clinical Nutrition* 40 (October 1984): 780–87.

Mellies, M. J., et al. "Effects of Varying Maternal Dietary Cholesterol and Phytosterol in Lactating Women and Their Infants." *American Journal of Clinical Nutrition* 37 (August 1978): 1347–54.

Finley, D. A., et al. "Food Choices of Vegetarians and Nonvegetarians During Pregnancy and Lactation." *Journal of the American Dietetic Association* 85 (June 1985): 678–85.

Fahraeus, L., O. Larrson-Cohn, and L. Wallentin. "Plasma Lipoproteins Including High Density Lipoprotein Subfractions During Normal Pregnancy." *Obstetrics and Gynecology* 66 (1985): 468–72.

Higginbottom, Sweetman, and Nyhan. "Syndrome in a Vitamin B_{12} Deficient Breastfed Infant." 317–23.

Bachrach, Fisher, and Parks. "Outbreak of Vitamin D Deficiency Rickets." 871–77.

Barber-Madden, R., M. A. Petschek, and J. Pakter. "Breastfeeding and the Working Mother: Barriers and Intervention Strategies." *Journal of Public Health Policy* 8 (1987): 531–41.

Gielen, A. C., et al. "Maternal Employment During the Postpartum Period: Effects on Initiation and Continuation of Breastfeeding." *Pediatrics* 87 (1991): 298–305.

INDEX

ABOUT THE AUTHOR

EILEEN BEHAN is a member of the American Dietetic Association, a registered dietitian, and a mother of two. She holds a degree in home economics from River College in Nashua, New Hampshire, and completed a traineeship in nutrition at Brigham and Women's Hospital in Boston. She has worked for the Harvard School of Public Health and the Veterans Administration, and for five years her show "Food for Talk" aired on Boston public radio. She currently works as a nutrition consultant, helping families to improve health through diet. She has also written *Microwave Cooking for Your Baby and Child* (Villard, 1991). She lives with—and feeds—her family in New Hampshire.